ALONE AND INVISIBLE NO MORE

*How Grassroots Community Action
and 21st Century Technologies Can
Empower Elders to Stay in Their Homes
and Lead Healthier, Happier Lives*

ALLAN S. TEEL, MD

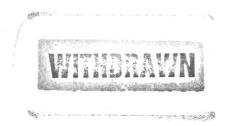

CHELSEA GREEN PUBLISHING
WHITE RIVER JUNCTION, VERMONT

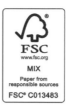
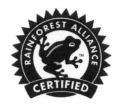

"This logo identifies paper that meets the standards of the Forest Stewardship Council.® FSC® is widely regarded as the best practice in forest management, ensuring the highest protections for forests and indigenous peoples."

Project Manager: Patricia Stone
Developmental Editor: Joni Praded
Copy Editor: Cannon LaBrie
Proofreader: Helen Walden
Designer: Peter Holm, Sterling Hill Productions

Printed in the United States of America
First printing June, 2011
10 9 8 7 6 5 4 3 2 1   11 12 13 14 15

green press INITIATIVE

Chelsea Green is committed to preserving ancient forests and natural resources. We elected to print this title on 30% post-consumer recycled paper, processed chlorine-free. As a result, we have saved:

15 Trees (40' tall and 6-8" diameter)
6 Million BTUs of Total Energy
1,519 Pounds of Greenhouse Gases
6,847 Gallons of Wastewater
434 Pounds of Solid Waste

Chelsea Green made this paper choice because our printer, Thomson-Shore, Inc., is a member of Green Press Initiative, a nonprofit program dedicated to supporting authors, publishers, and suppliers in their efforts to reduce their use of fiber obtained from endangered forests.

For more information, visit www.greenpressinitiative.org

Environmental impact estimates were made using the Environmental Defense Paper Calculator. For more information visit: www.edf.org/papercalculator

Our Commitment to Green Publishing

Chelsea Green sees publishing as a tool for cultural change and ecological stewardship. We strive to align our book manufacturing practices with our editorial mission and to reduce the impact of our business enterprise in the environment. We print our books and catalogs on chlorine-free recycled paper, using vegetable-based inks whenever possible. This book may cost slightly more because we use recycled paper, and we hope you'll agree that it's worth it. Chelsea Green is a member of the Green Press Initiative (www.greenpressinitiative.org), a nonprofit coalition of publishers, manufacturers, and authors working to protect the world's endangered forests and conserve natural resources. *Alone and Invisible No More* was printed on Natures Natural, a 30-percent postconsumer recycled paper supplied by Thomson-Shore.

Library of Congress Cataloging-in-Publication Data is available upon request.

Chelsea Green Publishing Company
Post Office Box 428
White River Junction, VT 05001
(802) 295-6300

www.chelseagreen.com

*To my family, friends, patients, and medical mentors
who have shared their wisdom and experiences with me.
May a new eldercare community honor their efforts.*

CONTENTS

ACKNOWLEDGMENTS

I now know why authors often take years to write a book. I also know why they are indebted to editors and friendly reviewers. I have so many to thank for helping this book get to print. Steve Larchuk insisted I write it and then helped me organize my often scattered thinking. Kim Fenn masterfully created the covers of the book's first version while providing encouragement when sorely needed. Carol Richards inspired many of the stories by working long hours treating every elder as a member of her family. Lexi Zoph, Jen Lacrosse, and Nikki Clifford gave A-plus dedicated service to members. Marie Fuller tried to keep me focused. Janet Yates, Roger Richards, Arthur Dexter, Sandra Lane, Sally Putonen, Judy Whitney, Carolyn Foster, and David Hinds volunteered mightily on behalf of our members. Frank Bedell, Carol Perry, Lila Blechman, Paige Stearns, Ella Mjelstad, Carolyn Howard, and Maria Del Carmen Yrbas Daneri helped out in many ways. David and Ceci Lampton, Sunil Rodrigues, Chris Pennock, Laurie Herron, Dorothy Petersen, Darrell Gudroe, John Hall, Jim Maxmin, Russ Lane, Chad Hanna, Dick Brown, and Meg Dexter invaluably shaped this elder model.

Now my new colleagues at Chelsea Green Publishing have stepped forward to help promote this project. I am grateful to have a publisher who shares my vision. Margo Baldwin immediately embraced the ideas. My editors Joni Praded and Cannon Labrie have made it a much better book. Pati Stone saw that it got out there.

My medical partners, Denise Soucy and Minda Gold, have been there for me for almost two decades. The ElderCare Network Board continues to work tirelessly to make "The Greens" prosperous. The nurses and staff of ElderCare Network, the Lincoln Home, and Cove's Edge shared their talents daily with my patients and me. Most importantly, so many older individuals entrusted me with their care, their wisdom, and their energy. It was their aspirations and their spirit that shaped all of the insights presented in this book.

My grown sons are a tremendous source of pride: Jon with his uncompromising honesty and Ben with his unwavering support. Deepest gratitude goes to my creative, dynamic, and charming wife, Carol Scales Teel, for showing me the way to truth and understanding. I alone take responsibility for any shortcomings in these chapters. I only hope that with time we can do justice to the legacy of so many older individuals who are a daily source of hope and inspiration to the rest of us.

INTRODUCTION

WHAT ARE WE DOING? We have segregated, isolated, and often marginalized a large group of older citizens who should be treated like celebrities at the later stages of their lives. In return for their sacrifice on our behalf, the rest of us have forgotten our elders and relegated them to a lonely existence often invisible to the community at large. While we honor sports figures with the Hall of Fame, actors with Lifetime Achievement Awards, and returning soldiers as national heroes, we neglect the millions of Americans who gave birth to us, built our communities, paid for the schools that educated us, and created many of the industries that sustain us. Many live in poverty today because they have outlived their savings. And now they are victims of a culture that worships youth and wealth, and ignores those who built the foundation for all we have.

The urgency of the situation is clear. As Shoshana Zuboff wrote in *Business Week,* "If health care is a train headed for a brick wall, then elder care is a high-speed train stuffed with our parents and grandparents racing toward a steel-reinforced concrete fortress. Today it's them. Tomorrow it's us." She concludes that "elder care as generally practiced is a euphemism for human warehousing on the cheap."[1]

Amen.

We had better change soon, because we are rapidly squandering our inheritance. We are wasting the resources older Americans discovered and created. Most importantly, we have chosen to push aside a generation that could contribute in so many ways with its wisdom, talent, and experience. Without a new, countrywide approach, the coming age wave's very numbers will soon swamp our financial and caregiver resources.

The projected demographics of aging America cannot be supported by our society's institutional infrastructure. The economics of our current approach—residential care in nursing homes and assisted-living homes—are unaffordable for most individuals, companies, insurance plans, and state and federal governments. Nearly every older individual and his or her family face the currently available options with dread or avoidance. With so much at stake, our leaders and our institutions procrastinate or continue to promote the same approach, hoping that doing the same thing over again will produce a different outcome.

In our political system, we have been debating the impending insolvency of Social Security since I was a high school student in the 1960s. Nearly fifty years later, we are no closer to having the political will to enact the necessary changes to fix the problem. Some national figures even question the wisdom of having any social safety net at all. Meanwhile, the urgency of addressing the fundamental needs of our elders increases incrementally each year.

I started medical school rather late in life, after having taught elementary school, and having worked in the building trades and the tourism industry. This varied background served me well as a family physician connecting with thousands of patients. I especially treasured my relationships with my older patients, as they shared their lives and their humanity with me. They taught me an enormous amount about what is important in life from their diverse experiences over their 70, 80, 90, even 100 years of living. My added training in geriatrics has sharpened my special focus on eldercare.

As the early chapters of this book reveal, I have seen up close every manner of institutional strategy employed to care for our aging population. I have done it all. I have provided eldercare in hospitals, at office visits, house calls, nursing homes, assisted-living residences, and in multigenerational households. I am the cofounder and president of our own ElderCare Network, a mini-system of seven small group homes in my Maine community that provide a more homelike experience for sixty elders who need daily services and support. Even though we have enjoyed some success with ElderCare Network, the handwriting is on the wall. I can see that simply doing institutional long-term care better will not solve the problems of cost and the human resources that are needed as tens of millions of baby boomers reach the age where increasing levels of support will be required.

Over my twenty-five years of medical practice, as I have contemplated the life stories of so many elders, and watched them pursue grossly inadequate options in the current health-care world, a comprehensive and radically different alternative eldercare model began to take shape in my mind.

With the help and sacrifice of many, my colleagues and I have brought those "better way" notions to life and call it, simply, the Maine Approach. It is a noninstitutional approach that enables even very frail elders, including those with fairly advanced memory loss, to remain at home at a fraction of the cost of institutional care.

"Eldercare" must also be redefined. Words—like "elder"—that signify age must not be used pejoratively. The vast majority of Americans now facing or long past retirement possess remarkable expertise that is often not valued, sought, or channeled in our communities. Most successful civilizations have revered their elders, and employed their wise counsel when charting future directions for their societies. The increasing disregard that our country displays for its most experienced members has not served us very well over the last fifty years, and worsens with each successive decade.

The implications of the word "care" are equally wrong. The current paradigm is about an external *us* defining the "care" for *them*. Too often their children and grandchildren, and the institutions that they delegate to make decisions on their behalf, define the terms of nearly all interactions with older individuals. Others then announce the plan, the schedule, the quality of life that older individuals are to embrace. By this method, we push our elders into a posture of denial or avoidance. We waste the opportunity to learn from their experiences and incorporate their knowledge into the decisions made, whether on a micro or macro level. How many of us even discuss what's going on in our personal and professional lives in any depth with our parents or our older friends and relatives? We have forgotten how to interact with our older community. We assume that they cannot contribute. Then we wonder why their lives and minds seem so dull.

Our elders are often hibernating, patiently waiting to be reengaged in living. We do not want to bother them. We forget they know a lot and probably faced a number of challenging circumstances at some point in their lives that are similar to our current concerns. Our elders do not want to bother us either, seeing how busy we are with our own lives. They do not want to butt in. They see and feel that they cannot perform with the same speed that they used to, so they back off, or are pushed aside, and quickly become invisible. The distance between the family and the community and our older individuals gets greater and greater. Initiatives like ours in Maine, if only on a small scale, reveal definitively that it does not have to be this way.

As you read about our Maine Approach in the pages ahead, you may find it shocking— perhaps even reckless. But before you judge too quickly or too harshly, ask yourself or ask an older member of your family this question: Is surviving the same as living? If your answer is that survival at all costs is all that matters, then my advice is to take this book back to where you purchased it and see if you can get a refund.

You see, with the Maine Approach we do not score successful aging by how many years we can stretch a life regardless of cost and regardless of the quality of those years. Rather we are committed to supporting our elders as they chart their own path.

We start with a commitment to help the elder members of our network live where they want to live. That usually means at home, however they may define it. And to do this we employ a combination of affordable high-technology monitoring devices, coordinated volunteer services, and a small committed core of skilled caregivers to deliver to each of our members—all elder-support clients—a customized bundle of support services wherever they call home.

Most importantly, we promote a very different attitude. We emphasize the importance of our elder clients finding a way to become involved in helping other elders. If we have a "secret sauce," this is it. Elder to elder, call it E2E if you like. And when it is blended with the right amount of high tech, organization, family, neighbors, and only as much skilled medical care as necessary, the results can be amazing.

Over the course of this book, I focus on how our community and our country cares for our elders and describe my personal path of discovery and frustration—which eventually leads to the development of the Maine Approach. With our approach, we currently care for over sixty members who are 80 to 104 years old and living happily at home. Our office manager is an unpaid retiree volunteer, as are most of the people in the organization. The cost to our members averages $400 per month, a small fraction of what they would expect to pay in an assisted-living facility or a nursing home. Many of our members are also my patients, and I can attest that there has been a dramatic reduction in the cost of emergency room and hospital care for those who have elected to leave institutional settings and return home. They have come full circle, and are better for it. And finally, our members are healthier and happier. Quite simply, they are living, not just surviving.

Of course the Maine Approach is not perfect. But by comparison with the alternative it is a quantum leap ahead of where we are and where we are headed. While actuaries and government planners may quibble over the exact numbers, there is no denying that a "gray tsunami" is headed our way. And we have already wasted too much time and money on a failed strategy of building more institutional and sterile warehouses for our elders.

If our success in Maine can be used as a model for millions of aging Americans, the overall reduction in health-care costs in the

United States can be significantly reduced without resort to rationing care and resources, or other unworkable approaches. That is why in the final chapters of the book I lay out a vision for transforming the way we can meet the challenge of tens of millions of elders, living longer, and rightfully demanding to be respected and to enjoy a role in their communities. National affiliates utilizing the Maine Approach and working through local physicians and local community organizations will be the vehicle to accomplish such an ambitious goal.

Government-run programs are not the answer. Even government-funded programs (if they survive the recession that persists as I write) must be designed with considerably less micromanagement and paper shuffling. Rather, this is a solution that will be driven from the grassroots, town by town and street by street. This effort must be done locally, driven by local community leaders, but with a national nongovernmental leadership.

In many cases, local family-practice physicians and dedicated nurses will take the lead, as nobody knows better the need for compassionate, affordable eldercare in their communities. As is, the current system is working against their practices—and their professions. The fiscal structure of the primary-care practice is not sustainable. In fact, the current payment system is scaring most current medical school students away from primary care, and pushing those in practice toward emergency room medicine, hospitalist medicine, or early retirement. Forecasts point to a primary-care physician shortage. Meanwhile, the specialist-laden system bankrupts state and federal coffers, as well as large and small businesses. Still we persist, digging the same hole faster and deeper instead of building a ladder. The Maine Approach will improve the efforts and economics of primary care physicians.

Religious institutions, home-health-care agencies, independent nurses, nurse practitioners, social workers, charity groups, foundations, schools, social organizations, even entrepreneurs such as disabled veterans or unemployed administrators can also become managers or cohosts of local organizations that can quickly grow and service dozens or even hundreds of elders who might otherwise have no choice but institutionalization.

To bring the Maine Approach to other communities across the nation over the next twenty years, we will need local chapters in every part of the country. This means a significant and meaningful employment opportunity for hundreds of thousands of people who will be doing very important work.

With a group of committed men and women I have founded a national organization—Full Circle America—to act as an umbrella and support center for those affiliates. With private funding from socially committed investors, we will provide local leaders with all of the tools they need to get started, even seed capital and training. Once a local affiliate is up and running, Full Circle America will be there to assume substantially all of the back-office administrative tasks, freeing the local manager to develop his or her volunteer base and help manage the local day-to-day operations.

Overall, the Maine Approach initiates an exciting transformation that provides a limitless talent pool to contribute to solving one of the most important problems our society faces. It effectively averts the economic disaster that "business as usual" will ensure. It will make all of us richer from the special relationships it champions. The framework for a powerfully effective solution to what seemed an intractable problem is right in front of us. It is up to us to see beyond the older faces and the slower gait. It requires us to venture out of our comfort zone a little. But the opportunities that such a different paradigm offers to all segments of society are boundless. Once you seriously consider such an approach, there is no going back. Anything less just won't do.

With tens of millions of older Americans in need we have no time to lose. If Facebook can go from nothing to 500 million members in five years, we can do this. And if we fail, we will have missed the opportunity to help save America from the financial and social crisis that is heading our way.

Thank you for your interest in this book and its ideas. I hope it will convince you that the challenge we face in dealing with an aging America is actually a test of our national character and an opportunity to excel as a people.

A quick note about the text: The names of some elders and others in these pages have been changed to protect their privacy. Many have proudly wanted their stories to be told and their names included. I have not changed the names of the ElderCare volunteers and support staff.

one

Gram Teel

HOW COULD GROWING UP next door to doting grandparents in a quiet suburban neighborhood not make the elder world attractive? Whether it was Gram's fresh cupcakes and her uniquely soft ice cream from her antique refrigerator, or collecting stamps with my grandfather on a warm summer Friday night in front of a black-and-white television and the floor fan, or independently exploring the drainage streams in their basement with our homemade toy boats after school—everything about my grandparents' home seemed all at once attractively quiet and orderly, curious, and supportive, full of treats and treasures in a very understated way. As I grew older and more consumed by my own pursuits, the appeal of time with them never diminished.

So when Gram turned ninety at her condo in Massachusetts and was driving my father crazy with her repetitious questions and stories, it seemed only natural to move her into an apartment near my wife and me in Maine. Because she wanted to have her cat with her, and wanted to maintain her independence as much as possible, institutional care was not an option. She was still driving despite barely seeing over the dashboard, and her car was an essential part of her self-sufficiency. She never had an accident, and never got lost. At McDonald's, she would eat inexpensively, and introduce herself to each new acquaintance as simply "Gram." At home, she would focus on feeding her huge cat, Jack, a gift from a grandchild, and would occasionally play rough enough to have bruised and scratched forearms, but would never let you utter a critical word about Jack, or about anyone for that matter.

Despite her quiet manner, she would occasionally let you in on her many secrets. Once while I was in my twenties, when we were talking about life in general and about my parents' divorce in particular, I marveled at how she had been happily married for almost fifty years. She quietly said, "It wasn't always easy you know. . . ." No further elaboration. That was as close to a complaint as I ever heard from her. That was often the way her generation approached such delicate issues.

And for her, it had not always been easy. Although growing up as the oldest child in an upper-middle-class family, she was so painfully shy that she could not attend school regularly. Having outgoing younger siblings did not help. As an adult, her third child was born just as the stock market crashed and her father's bank failed. Gram then raised her family during the depression, as did so many of her generation. Much later she faced the last twenty-five years of her life alone after my grandfather, a nonsmoker, died of lung cancer in his late sixties.

Gram taught me a lot about successful aging. After Gramp's death, she continued as the reliable friend and taxi for many of her former neighbors who then lived in the area's senior apartment complexes. As fewer and fewer of her friends drove, she became busier. Gram derived great satisfaction and sense of purpose from her role in their lives. She took many to lunch and to their appointments.

Her community service had started much earlier. Her father had funded and her mother had administered the Home for the Aged in Reading, Massachusetts. After her kids were grown, Gram was appointed its president, and as my dad said, "She really got her teeth into it."

There she found her voice, and effectively advocated for and cared for its residents until the home closed in the 1960s with the advent of a local nursing home. From my preschool days, I have vague memories of being exposed to the world of isolated rooming-house elders. So in many ways, it seems that taking an advocacy role for elders is in my blood.

From the time I first noticed, Gram never seemed in a hurry. She moved at a tempered pace and yet never seemed to waste a step. She did not have unattainable expectations. She was flexible enough to roll with the opportunities that presented themselves on a regular basis. Pets were very important. She always had a dog or a cat, usually fed the wild birds by throwing breadcrumbs out the back door, or tended a parakeet. Even looking at horses in a pasture could light up her face. When she was driving by, she would often pull over for a moment to watch. We would often wonder how she could get her car so dirty!

Her car was critical because she no longer walked as far or as steadily as she used to. Her trips were short and often were an excuse to just get out of the house. Often, she would meet someone new at a diner or a sandwich shop. As she grew older, she met new people easily, and especially liked young people. They bonded immediately with very few words spoken.

Loneliness was her biggest lament. She never had enough visitors. She loved to hear from her family, but she preferred them to visit and bring their children, or their friends, and photographs, and tell her about their latest projects. It did not matter what time of day or night any of us arrived at her apartment. She was always waiting for us, and excited to cater to us. Food and hospitality went hand in hand. Each visitor was offered a cookie, a cupcake, a sandwich, or a cup of coffee. Gram always treated our friends as one of the family—making everyone comfortable in an easy chair or at the kitchen table.

She continued this pattern even when my wife and I moved her to Maine, near us, in her nineties. Gram befriended an emotionally challenged young woman who lived alone in the low-income housing complex to which she had moved. She often ran errands for her or even loaned her a few dollars. She was enormously open and trusting, and to my knowledge was never burned by her approach.

She appreciated her independence and at the same time trusted that things would work out. Once when she slid to the floor near her bed in the wee morning hours, she pulled the bedclothes down around her to be warm and made do until the cleaning lady arrived. Why bother someone by pushing her lifeline button?

Gram went to bed shortly after supper, and she rarely got up at night, and never had to change bedding unnecessarily. She was one of the lucky ones. It is curious in this time of technically complex medical care how important it is to have good bladder control to maintain one's independence and not be placed in residential care owing to urinary incontinence. We have made this issue one of the triggers leading to institutionalization even though a change in venue does not solve the problem. This is an example of how concern about one very specific trigger can blind family and health-care decision-makers to an elder's overall enjoyment of life. In a not so distant past, extended families lived near each other, and frequent intergenerational contact was the norm. Family relationships were often very fluid, and visits quite informal. In my case, it was commonplace to be instructed to go to Gram's house after school. Most importantly, very few members of the older generation were isolated. Many days while growing up, I remember my grandmother's Uncle Fred perched at his workbench under the apple tree in our backyard, and his black Model T parked in Gram's driveway next door. He was often busy carving some small item for his complex dioramas, when one of our errant baseballs landed near his spot in our short left field. We would even draw him into umpiring a close call from time to time. His life in his declining years still had purpose and connections.

Even as twenty-first-century life has become more complicated, and the key issues of aging get more technical and the approaches to them become more institutionalized, most of what is important in day-to-day life is still nonmedical: staying connected to family, friends, and lifelong interests. Community is important. Remaining independent keeps one healthier. Having a purpose, whether it is caring for a pet, or participating in the life of an extended family or a neighbor, is essential. No matter what our age, we need a reason to get up in the morning. We feel much better when we do something for others, and by extension, doing for others keeps us mentally and physically healthier. Worrying is unhealthy, and solves very few problems. Intergenerational connections are vital to reducing loneliness and isolation and provide extraordinary mutual benefit.

So much of my thinking in the movement to revolutionize eldercare as we know it is shaped by Gram and her simple principles. This graceful, matter-of-fact woman, and many others like her, understood their own needs and fulfilled them in part by embracing and serving others in true community. Revisiting her story is not a wistful exercise in nostalgia; rather it is a blueprint for a better way.

two

The Gray Tsunami

GRAM TEEL WAS LIKE SO many other quintessential grandmothers. We can all identify with her character. She was able to live independently in her own home or apartment surrounded by her familiar furnishings and memories of her lifetime until the week before she died. She was able to care for her beloved cat, and entertain family and friends regularly, on her own terms, in her own environment. Such an outcome should not be rare or so difficult to achieve. Yet it is.

In chapter 3, we will review the last century of residential-care options for elders. It will be painfully clear that there has never been a heyday for eldercare. To date there has not been an appealing, reasonable solution. It is quite easy to criticize many features in the previous and current options that we as a community dislike or even detest. It is quite another thing to assemble a workable, affordable alternative.

I will also share with you my personal history in the eye of the gathering storm—providing an inside look at a typical nursing home and some assisted-living homes to provide some vantage point on their scope of care, to let you see a few of the elders, and a few of the issues that surround those facilities. We will explore the regulatory challenges that frustrate all attempts to create a more workable solution.

Before going there, however, and to focus the mind a bit, we need to invest in some shock therapy, to understand the demographic trends that are currently upon us. The current and future financial implications of the way we presently do elder residential care are self-evident and undeniable. Business as usual is not an option. We cannot afford it. And frankly, no one wants it.

So before we begin to shape that better option, let us look closely, in bullet-point fashion, at the facts and scope of the demographic and economic challenges that an aging U.S. population poses for the entire country. Just over the horizon is truly a gray tsunami:

- In 2008, 35 million Americans were over age 65.
- By 2020, this figure will grow to 55 million.
- By 2030, 85 million Americans will be over age 65.
- The fastest growing segment of the population is those over 85.
- Over 4 million are over 85 now.
- By 2050 an estimated 21 million will be over 85.
- There will be 1 million Americans over age 100 by 2050.
- Current life expectancy for the average 65-year-old is twenty years.
- Half of all Americans over 65 are admitted to a nursing home at least once.
- Nursing homes currently serve 1.5 million.
- Twenty-two percent of all Americans over 85 live in institutional settings.
- Forty percent of elderly women and 20 percent of elderly men currently live at home alone.
- Twenty million American families have an individual older than 80 living with them.
- There are 6.9 million Americans working as long-distance caregivers.
- Waiting lists for home-based services in thirty-one states exceed 300,000.
- In 1943, the United States had 43 working people for each retiree. By 2015 it will be 2.

- By 2030 one-third of the adult population will be over 65.
- The estimated caregiver shortage by 2030 will be 20 million.

Every one of these statistics speaks to the need to do something urgently about our impending aging tidal wave. You cannot pick up a magazine or newspaper without seeing a story that adds another grim fact about our aging population.

The financial aspects of the aging crisis are even more worrisome:

- Nursing home costs for a single elder in the northeastern United States now exceed $100,000 per year.
- Assisted-living fees routinely exceed $60,000 per year.
- Around-the-clock, in-home, private care can exceed $175,000 per year.
- Institutional care expenses are rising much faster than the general rate of inflation.
- Only 1 percent of Americans can afford to self-pay these costs.
- Most elders are routinely and quickly bankrupted by these charges.
- Bankrupt elders end up on state Medicaid rolls.
- Especially in recessionary times states cannot carry this burden.
- Despite the increasing demand, many institutional residential-care facilities are going out of business due to the inability of their patients to pay for care and the failure of state government to increase Medicaid reimbursements to keep up with inflation.
- Construction of more residential-care facilities will deplete government resources required to support other public infrastructure. In my thinly populated

county in Maine, unless we change our strategy for dealing with our aging population, we will require over 500 more institutional units and care by 2030. This will impose an average *annual* tax cost per household of $5,000.

- Annual health-care expenditures in the United States exceed $2.5 trillion, a staggering 16 percent of our gross domestic product, and growing toward 30 percent by 2050.
- Even with a Medicare outlay of more than $300 billion per year, 95 percent of those over 65 live at home and receive very little financial or personal assistance from government—a foreboding prospect as we anticipate tripling the number of Americans over 65 years old in the next twenty years.

Whether we use local, state, or federal numbers, the population distribution is drastically changing, and not at some distant future date. It is upon us now and will continue to worsen yearly, for the next forty years. The economics of addressing this gray tsunami with the approaches we are using now will not work. Worse, because the crisis has already begun, we do not have the luxury of planning for this eventuality for a decade or two and budgeting for such changes.

This is not a situation where we just need to tweak or fine-tune the institutional residential system we have been using for some sixty years. There is simply not enough money to do so. Future chapters describe our own heartbreaking efforts in Maine to make a noninstitutional residential-care approach a financially viable solution. Nor can we spare from the ever-shrinking younger workforce the millions of men and women that will be required to provide paid day-to-day care for our elder population.

Fortunately, there are solutions that are within our reach, utilizing existing human, financial, and technological resources. But it will take a lot of education and cultural change to accomplish them.

The solution we have developed over the last five years in midcoast Maine—the Maine Approach—follows these cardinal principles drawn from analyzing the above statistics:

- Business as usual is not an option. No county, state, or federal governments, no private companies, and not many private individuals can afford either the financial or human-resource costs of the current residential-care model of eldercare when it is expanded to meet the demographic needs of the baby boomers.
- The health-care system as we know it is irreparably broken and financially unsustainable. Major reform still seems far away.
- The prospect of housing millions more people in to-be-built new residential homes is not feasible, or even desirable.
- We need to totally rethink what we are doing, and the way we do it.
- As social entrepreneurs on many fronts are highlighting, we cannot just reduce cost; we need to create new sources of value and tap new sources of service, support, and advice.
- The future elder consumers will not be as tolerant as the current cohort. Moreover, they have not saved as frugally, and the workforce to support them will be dramatically smaller.
- We must put the needs of the individual, not the institution, at the center.
- Elders are segregated, isolated, and undervalued. Retirement communities and residential-care facilities take our valuable elder resource out of circulation.
- We need to rebuild community trust and dignity again for our elders. Successful civilizations from

the beginning of recorded history have valued their
elders.
• Change will require serious effort from many
sectors. To paraphrase a well-known saying, it will
take a village to care for our elders. The impending
age wave is not going to be gentle—it is more of a
tsunami. Urgent action is demanded.

The cornerstones of the Maine Approach are utilizing web-based
technology tools alongside volunteer and paid staff—from the elder
cohort itself, as well as from the rest of the community—to help the
vast majority of elders who so desire to remain at home and more
connected to family, friends, personal interests, and community.

It is a Gram Teel lifestyle with a modern twist. The Maine
Approach has shown us that it is possible to reconnect elders with
their communities, families, and caregivers and help them live independently. We do this by offering robust social networking, life-
management tools, and video-monitoring technology, along with
check-ins and a broad suite of services delivered by staff and volunteers. It taps a huge hidden resource of capable elders to address the
tasks that need doing to keep elders in their own homes—from telephone calls to video calls to hosting other elders to providing rides to
delivering meals to home visits. It reconfigures existing community
assets like schools, churches, and existing community businesses to
support this elder network. It promotes a much more individualized
approach than is possible in institutional residential care. It values
independence and interdependence, while giving each elder lasting
purpose and meaning in his or her life.

And the cost? About *10 percent* of what we are paying now for a
failing and unsustainable system. Later chapters describe in detail
what we learned and how America can very quickly ramp up to
adopt the Maine Approach in every neighborhood.

• three •

A Brief History of
Residential Care in America

I ARRIVED IN DAMARISCOTTA, MAINE, in 1988, fresh out of a high-quality, very challenging family-practice residency at Lancaster General Hospital in Pennsylvania. I was to take over a busy, well-established family practice, and I could not have been more excited.

Before meeting the moving van, my family stopped downtown at the Salt Bay Café for some lunch. As luck would have it, an older woman tripped on the uneven grade into the restaurant and nearly fell in my lap. Unfortunately for her, her left foot was now externally rotated indicating a likely broken hip. She became my first admission to the hospital. My career of integrating geriatric care into my everyday life in this community had begun.

Some of my older patients resided at the Lincoln Home in Newcastle, Maine, and soon after my arrival, I became its medical director—a position I would hold for fifteen years. The Lincoln Home was a grand riverside private home opened as a "home for the aged" in 1932 through local benefactors. The home's history illustrates the history of residential care for elders in America.

Homes for the aged, as they were called, began in the early twentieth century as a part of the social activism of many newly formed women's groups that had also adopted temperance and voting rights among their better-remembered causes.

In many cases, these homes were a reaction to the poor farms and almshouses that many communities had established in the late 1800s. The almshouses functioned as human warehouses, or a sort of rudimentary welfare system for everyone that did not fit in: the insane, the poor, the homeless, the derelicts, older orphans, elders without family. Gradually, various charitable organizations, often with either immigrant or religious roots, formed to take certain subgroups out of this mix and take care of them separately in specially designated homes.

These actions caused a dramatic change in the makeup of the resident population in the almshouses. As reported and described by social historian Carole Haber:

> In 1880, 33 percent of the almshouse population was composed of elderly individuals; but by 1923, the proportion had increased to 67 percent. . . . In New York City, in 1903, the Charity Board renamed its public almshouse the Home for the Aged and Infirm. . . .
>
> Despite the name changes and the rosy descriptions that filled the institutions' annual reports, most people hardly looked upon the almshouse as a satisfactory solution to the demands for long-term care for the elderly. Throughout the early twentieth century, the institution remained a symbol of failure and despair.[1]

So almshouses and poor farms had evolved into de facto elder housing, better than nothing and less problematic given the shorter life expectancy of the times.

It was in this era of social activism and reexamination that the Lincoln Home was founded in Maine. In 1925, Lillian Nash, whose husband owned the first telephone company in the area, took her idea to secure a home for elderly people in Lincoln County to a joint meeting of seven women's clubs at the Cavanaugh House in Damariscotta Mills, Maine, as guest of the Magazine Club. After hearing the presentation, each club put up one dollar to seal its commitment, and the project was on.

Over the next few years, a Union of Women's Clubs was formed, then incorporated. Bylaws were written, a board of directors elected, a suitable place for their home for the aged was found. Monies were raised, and renovations began. The first four residents, along with their caretaker/matron husband-and-wife team, moved into the remodeled twenty-room house in late 1932. Even Frances Perkins, Franklin Roosevelt's secretary of labor with local roots, and Maine governor Tudor Gardiner attended the opening of the Lincoln Home. In the worst days of the worst depression in American history, local commitment with local private funds and ingenuity had made one person's dream a reality.

For nearly sixty years, the Lincoln Home continued to serve a vital role in the community, providing communal living for older persons in relatively good health. Women's clubs projects and charitable giving funded any unmet financial needs. Members were encouraged to remember the Lincoln Home in their wills, with these bequests helping form the Lincoln Home Endowment. The home accepted residents who had limited assets, and committed to care for them for the rest of their lives. New residents turned over whatever they had in return for life tenancy. As houses had little value during the Depression, this was considered a good exchange.

From its inception, the focus was on a homelike atmosphere, emphasizing the "friendliness of the staff, the smells of something good cooking in the kitchen, private rooms with private baths, and pleasant common living and dining rooms."[2] The concept and execution was anything but institutional. No mention was made of health qualifications or of financial exclusions for elders seeking admission.

The politics and financial realities of long-term care then as now were never far below the surface. Many communities were accused of keeping public-assistance housing substandard so as not to encourage its growth. In the early days before Social Security, some leaders favored a pension for the elderly instead of supported housing. Once Social Security was passed, in an effort to empty out the almshouses, federal legislation in the 1930s barred any resident from receiving the recently enacted "old-age support." However, elderly residents of private homes for the aged could receive their old-age pension. So, of course, over the next twenty years, most government-sponsored almshouses and poor farms disappeared and were replaced by new homes for the aged.

Policy makers and pension advocates of the day both had over-looked the physical health needs of many older residents. In a time when the average life expectancy barely reached sixty years, many believed that with a small guaranteed annuity individuals could live independently. Conversely, Homer Folks, an aging advocate of the time, observed that most older individuals in almshouses were there because of a medical necessity that required a hospital or nurs-ing facility of some sort. It was not just their poverty. This debate presaged the central theme that continues today about how we address the social, holistic needs of a rapidly growing elder popula-tion, while not ignoring their concomitant medical needs.

As homes for the aged proliferated rapidly, another critical issue overlooked was finding a balance between regulatory oversight and the unscrupulous greed of some private business owners. In 1960, the Lincoln Home was filled to capacity when it faced its own regula-tory battle. It was "dealt a heavy blow" by Maine legislation requir-ing sprinkler systems for such homes, even though the logistics of getting water to the third-floor bedrooms of the Lincoln Home were impractical.

The home responded to that regulation with a major building campaign, also hoping to shorten its long waiting list. Many of the same dedicated community members from the area women's clubs that were instrumental in the founding of the Lincoln Home also led the new fund-raising effort. It culminated in an annex opening in 1964. Still, the primary focus of the Lincoln Home was comfortable surroundings and good fellowship.

On a national level, alternating waves of scandal and regulation appeared. In 1954, in an attempt to raise the quality of elder residen-tial care, and to address the enormous backlog of need in almost every community, the Hill-Burton Hospital Survey and Construction Act was passed. It provided federal grants for the construction of nursing homes that were affiliated with a hospital.

Following the inevitable theme of building what can be funded, many new nursing homes were built as an integrated part of acute-care hospitals. The move transferred the nursing home from being a part of the despised welfare system to part of the health-care system. This evolution was to be a mixed blessing.

By 1960, major nursing home scandals were widely reported, cataloging financial irregularities, uncovering poor staffing, and illuminating inadequate adherence to code and regulation. By 1968, Congress passed comprehensive legislation to improve nursing homes with the Moss Amendment. However, most nursing homes were unable to comply with the new standards owing to cost constraints, and, in 1971, the Miller Amendment lowered standards of care to affordable levels.

In the mid-1970s, scandals involving provider fraud and poor care again broke out across the country. It is no wonder most of my elder patients fear the thought of being placed in a nursing home. They had lived through several well-publicized accounts of substandard conditions in many such facilities.

Few additional national changes occurred until 1985 when the Institute of Medicine published its landmark report on nursing home care. That report led to the Omnibus Reconciliation Act of 1987, which produced the largest overhaul of federal nursing home regulations ever undertaken. Almost immediately, the number of nursing homes grew rapidly, as did Medicare expenditures on them. Then the Balanced Budget Act of 1997 went in the other direction and significantly cut the amount of money Medicare paid nursing homes.[3] Within two years, this event triggered four large nursing home chains to declare bankruptcy.

This brief recap of a century of changes in elder residential care allows us to see the political ambivalence that has existed toward eldercare for a long time. It does not appear that any policy maker ever foresaw nursing homes as the primary residential-care option for our elders. Nursing homes have become this by default. For most of their existence, residential-care facilities were seen as the best option for those who had no choice. They were not the preferred way of addressing elder issues. And over the course of the twentieth century, as the population over 65 grew from 3 million to 35 million, the challenges of addressing elder issues comprehensively have mushroomed.

Initially homes for the aged were conceptually simple: room and board in a community home; meals served family style; boarders coming and going as they chose; stairways to navigate; very few rules; some volunteer labor and maybe a paid staff person; no regulations; and started by the generosity of some town fathers or town mothers who recognized the need to provide some dignity and normalcy for a few isolated local elders.

The current reality is that nursing homes and assisted-living facilities run the gamut from luxurious to the barely tolerable. Those privileged few who can afford the most posh can enjoy a near-resort experience with gourmet meals, low staff-to-resident ratios, organized recreational and educational activities, and all with trained medical staff at the ready.

For the vast majority of older Americans the experience is much different. While most of these facilities are staffed by underpaid individuals attempting to provide the very best experience they can within ever-diminishing budgets, the simple fact is that time, and money, is running out.

I have many older patients who will not even set foot in a residential-care facility. One refers to the local nursing home as "the Big House," a prison reference that says it all. Many fear that a "visit" will quickly become the loss of home and independence. I am not sure that I blame them. But with the Maine Approach as a model, we can all do better.

• four •

The Lincoln Home

THE LINCOLN HOME STILL SERVES elders in my community—and represents one major facet of residential care there. While it began as a home for the aged, it has been extensively reengineered as a private assisted-living facility with a few elder apartments in the last decade. It is at the Lincoln Home where we can put a human face on the changes elders have faced in the last few decades. When I first came to town in the 1980s, much like the previous fifty years, one's day-to-day needs at the Lincoln Home were nicely met by a small staff of dedicated caregivers, long on common sense and often without formal training or credentials.

Ella, Annette, and Faylene knew all the residents' needs and their life stories. They were very ably supervised by a very bright, very organized, nonmedical neighbor-administrator. The home thrived, still fulfilling the very valuable mission for the county envisioned by its founders.

Clara Storm and her husband Alex moved into the Lincoln Home in the 1960s in their sixties—and their story epitomizes the standard of care in that era. Despite Alex's roots in German prewar nobility, Clara was in charge but deferential. Always practical, she saw early on that the time was coming when they would need help, as they were childless and an ocean away from any other relatives. They were also too far from her business-career roots in New York City. The benefits of group living that the Lincoln Home offered effectively self-insured them against the unpredictable events of aging, and allowed them to stay in the community they now called home.

Clara was a large woman with a thick accent who astutely observed everything at the home, and gently and diplomatically shaped much that went on around her. She also gave back by writing a column for over thirty years for the area weekly newspaper, the *Lincoln County News*. She remained active in the community and was a formidable ambassador for the home throughout her entire stay there. When the board of trustees suggested a founders' day auction to help fund operating expenses at the home, *resident* Clara Storm, not a board member, was the person who volunteered to lead the effort. That auction continues today.

Although Clara never expected to live to be 100, she did. Yet in her last few years, despite deep-seated affection for the Lincoln Home, she could not help commenting on the changes being implemented at the end of her watch. A multimillion dollar renovation gave her luxurious living quarters that she loved to show off, but the personality of the place had grown different too, and she did not like that change of character.

Layers of staff, all licensed, documented their charts well, but did not have the time or inclination to sit with the residents on the porch or in the backyard. The previous unlicensed regular staff was kept on and retrained by state licensing authorities as this transition took place. Though they still retained their personal connections to many older residents, their insights and experience were often underutilized by the newer, institutionally trained staff, and certainly unappreciated by the state regulators.

The new institutional environment was dominated by professional RN administrators and certified medication passers; communications between health-care colleagues were limited only to signed faxes; telephone orders between doctor and nonprofessional staff were no longer allowed. Trips to the emergency room also became much more frequent. Strict adherence to state regulations meant always acting defensively, always in preparation for the next state inspection. Common sense and improvisation were not valued commodities. Spontaneity was infrequent. Clara would have definitely given us an earful.

Financing had also dramatically changed. Promises to care for residents for the rest of their lives were no longer possible. Exploding health-care costs had outstripped the resources of the previously successful and sensible approach of the founders. Despite the desire to meet the needs of a diverse area population, with private-pay monthly costs running $5,000–$6,000 per resident, decisions needed to be shaped by financial realities.

Of course, the Lincoln Home is not alone. The entire eldercare landscape has changed. Each resident has very different and vastly more complicated medical needs. Family expectations have also changed as the costs have increased. Whereas residents and their families were once satisfied with a clean, well-maintained room and wholesome meals, today, assisted-living facilities must provide very much more. The medical culture has created a complex system of assisted living based on a nursing home model where the frequent checking of vital signs, the administration of lots of pills and shots at specific times, regular lab tests and doctors' office visits, emergency-room evaluations in the middle of the day and night, and close supervision of residents during every part of every day, have become the norm.

Assisted-living facilities have become the step-down unit, or poor stepchild, of the nursing facility. Modest assistance has grown into extraordinary assistance. Independent-living apartments are actually an oxymoron. No one residing within these walls is truly independent. There are just varying degrees of dependency. And the current environment fosters more dependency.

Arlene's story typifies much of this new era. An artist by training who taught at the college level in Rhode Island, she has always been fiercely independent by nature. She moved into the Lincoln Home about five years ago in her early nineties—not on her own initiative, but at the insistence of her doctor and her lawyer owing to *their* concerns about her failing eyesight. She regularly reminds any listener that moving there really was not her idea. She would rather be home. She did not have any real choice. This was not the way Clara Storm and her generation came to live there.

Although Arlene's basic needs are nicely covered at the Lincoln Home, she begrudgingly acknowledges that most days she would rather have the capricious, unpredictable, and even risky existence of living in a less-controlled environment. She rolls her eyes at the regulatory redundancy. She gravitates to the common-sense-driven staff holdovers from the earlier era. She concludes most of her complaints with a refrain, "What do you expect from me, I'm old."

I believe that the reduced choice and lack of personal control that institutional living delivers compounds the bitterness that many individuals come to feel when trying to cope with the physical disabilities that often accompany advanced aging. At 92, Arlene has as good a mind as any I have known. Yet she has developed a sharper tongue with age, something that probably stems from missing the sensitivity and human interactions that characterized most of her earlier life. Her badly declining vision colors her mood profoundly. However, she retains her ability to see clearly what is going on, and to know that it is not right.

Arlene is just feisty enough to regularly question authority, "What are they going to do to me at my age?" When given the opportunity, she flashes the smile and the sparkle from those earlier times. She hangs on to control whenever she can, even if it is only ordering medications herself from Walmart rather than having the residential home take over that function too.

She is a good analyst on the inside of this institution. A smart reformer or administrator would do well to listen to her.

Having been in the middle of this transformation from "homes for the aged" to the appearance of "assisted living," I realized long ago that we have sacrificed many vitally important elements along the way. We have seen regulatory policy trump common sense. We have watched medical concerns overwhelm human needs. We have seen cost limit choice and determine eligibility. More recently, we have learned that many elders admitted to these institutions do not need to be there. Rather, they can and should be in their own individual homes or in *Golden Girls*–style shared homes with as much support as they need. This is the Maine Approach, and it works.

• five •

Cove's Edge

THE OTHER MAJOR ARM of residential care in my community has been the nursing home. We have seen how the Lincoln Home assisted-living facility has struggled to hold its course in stormy seas. Similarly, our local nursing homes have been battered despite the best efforts of all involved.

In the 1980s, the Miles Memorial Hospital "nursing facility" was housed on the top floor of the hospital, as promoted by the Hill-Burton legislation of the 1950s. Long-term care was essentially crowded double rooms without a lot of extras. A few of the more mobile residents could visit a tiny solarium at the end of the hall. The routine was very basic: meals and most of your life spent in a double room divided by a curtain. Nurses administered your medications and would troubleshoot problems as well as size up your personality. It certainly felt like an extension of the hospital below, as its funding legislation intended.

In the early 1990s, the Miles campus planned for a new nursing home, and I became the medical director for the new Cove's Edge Nursing Facility. New construction brought dramatic changes: more light and more space: vaulted ceilings with atrium-delivered natural lighting; a large living room with a big-screen television; an activity room; wide hallways, patio space, a hair salon, and whirlpool; dining options fed by an expansive commercial kitchen. All these represented a dramatic departure from the cramped physical space that had existed before.

But the patient rooms were still double rooms separated by

a curtain with a bath shared among four residents. The windows were bigger, but the closets were small, and the space allowed only a bureau and an easy chair. How much progress had we really made?

The professionalization of the entire process of residential care also came with the new facility. There was a distinct administrative wing separated by limited-access double doors. There were staff break rooms and charting rooms efficiently removed from the bustle of residents' activities. Nurses' stations with security alarms and window walls enabled staff to keep an eye on residents while doing the burgeoning paperwork.

It was all so seductively institutional.

Dedicated long-term caregivers from RNs to certified nursing aides (CNAs) still patrolled the halls, befriended the elders that moved into the facility, and consoled their families. But more nursing time was spent tied to medication carts, faxing memos to doctors' offices, and addressing concerns of dietary consultants, pharmacy consultants, wound-care consultants, as well as the ever-expanding documentation requirements for reimbursement. Activities and true human interaction became the designated job of the activity director, and the occasional province of the unit secretary who often became the only regular employee in the traffic pattern of pleasantly demented residents moving about the facility. Human touch was harder to come by, and continued to get scarcer every year.

Of course the dedicated nurses and aides that worked there were still to be commended. During the early days, administrator Linda and head nurses Carolyn and Nancy constantly connected with all the residents under their supervision. They were rarely in their offices, preferring to be mixing it up with the residents, sharing the joys and sadness, the wonder and pace of every day in the lives of this fragile cohort. Similarly, RNs Dawn, Saima, and Carol and a few other key nurses were a wealth of inside information on all the residents on their wings, and clearly acted like an extended family member with all of them. The love reciprocated by the most difficult residents made it all worthwhile for them.

However, these old-school nurses were anachronistic—throwbacks to a previous era. As paperwork and other duties mounted, caregivers were increasingly distanced from the residents. Year after year, they have been beaten down by an administrative system that does not value the essence of what is and should be important in the lives of the residents of the nursing home: human connections. They understood the needs of elders because they had spent time with them, observing and listening, and truly caring. Many have left Cove's Edge rather than watch the atmosphere decline further.

This is not to say that the majority of the staff now function in an impersonal way. Quite the contrary. Bits of humor and true compassion are a part of nearly every shift there. Staff could not survive otherwise. But these interactions happen because the people that go into health care in general, and nursing home care in particular, do so because they are remarkably caring individuals who are enormously dedicated to the people they serve.

Such personal interactions do not happen because the institution fosters them. As a matter of fact, the regulatory environment insists that the nursing home stay clear of deficiencies and abuse, and often not much more. When you mention socialization or a holistic approach to the state or federal bureaucrats, you are labeled as a heretic or worse. To meet the needs and desires of nursing-home residents will require major cultural change.

Jenelle is another staff person that "gets it," and in my opinion is probably the best activity director in the entire state of Maine. She has defined her own role, and fashioned a schedule at great personal sacrifice that has her working afternoons, nights, and especially weekends, when there are few administrative types or nine-to-five medical and therapy professionals available. It is during these unofficial hours that she can work her magic of engaging elders in more purposeful activities. She regularly gathers a group of ladies around her in the spare kitchen at 8:00 PM after others have been tucked in. Together they make s'mores and tell stories about first loves and old boyfriends. She organizes performances by storytellers and musicians. Mostly, she reaches out to residents, learning about their lives, their personalities, their interests. On weekends, she often takes a wheelchair-bound resident for a walk, or to the coffee shop across the street for an ice cream. Sunshine and fresh air matter.

One time, Jenelle corralled me into taking four men down to the bridge in the center of Damariscotta to fish, and promptly left me there. With fishing lines in the river, an O'Doul's on the railing in front of each of their wheelchairs, and the sun shining brightly, it was a glorious afternoon. When Jenelle was out of sight, we decided to play a joke on her. I went into the nearby fish market and got a large frozen halibut and attached it to Merle's line. Because of his short-term memory problems, he promptly forgot it was there. When Jenelle returned, I exhorted him to reel it in, and he exuberantly went to work. A few minutes later, he proudly showed off his trophy fish. He then brought it back to the nursing home, and Jenelle made sure he and his buddies shared it for supper. Efforts like hers that should be applauded loudly and made commonplace stand out because they are so infrequent.

Most of the nursing home activity surrounds pill administration as well as required tasks such as controlled-substance reassessments, consultations such as skin integrity checks, confirming mandated order renewals, completing mental-health status forms, mandated doctor-office notifications of falls or brief changes in status. More and more documentation is tied to the reimbursement triggers of the state and federal scoring system. More and more of the direct care is delegated to the least experienced members of the health-care team, the newly hired aides. These young people are underpaid and all too quickly burn out, leading to rapid turnover and lack of continuity of care.

At the nursing home, residents are loved, dressed, and fed. But the rest of the time goes slowly—parked in wheelchairs alone in the corridors, in the courtyard, or in front of the television. Young people rarely appear on the premises, except when Christmas caroling. And when they do come by, many seem awkward and uncomfortable as they've had such little contact with older patients. Music, storytelling, and just plain human interaction are too infrequent and take a distant second place to other medical aspects of the day. Visits from family and friends are much too rare.

Yet an aging population housed within the nursing facility has no *medical* issue too small that there cannot be a remedy sought or a program initiated. Each new therapist will valiantly seek to address a resident's chronic problem with a newer appliance or drug and the accompanying documentation forms to ensure payment. They are unaware of and unable to decipher prior attempts that were made to solve the same problem because the answers are often buried in volumes of paper stored in another part of the building. The increasingly rapid evaluation of any potential acute medical problem means most nursing home residents will live in this purgatory for many years. And thus mere survival is the bureaucratic equivalent of living—a low standard but one easy to score.

Ida's story vividly illustrates these challenges. At 83, she has already resided in nursing homes for more than six years. After her husband died, and her confusion and dementia worsened, living at home was no longer thought to be safe. She nearly burned down her home by starting a fire on the porch. Her subsequent strokes and Parkinsonism caused profound stiffness and contractures of her limbs and neck. She spends most waking hours reclined in a gerichair in her room in a contorted position with her limbs shaking, and staring straight ahead while country music videos and game shows emanate from the TV on her dresser. She is tough to communicate with and even tougher to observe in these final stages of her diseases.

Recently, however, I took a few minutes to just sit beside her and try to find out what she was thinking. My first four or five questions did not produce any response at all. Then I asked, "Is there something that troubles you the most?" Without hesitation she replied, "Loneliness," unable to control her drooling as she said it. I was stunned. "I don't see you out of your room very often. Is that because you don't like the way you look?" I pressed on. "I just can't do what I used to anymore," she clearly stated. Another long pause. As I commented on the country music, and asked about music in her life, she shared a few details about her mother, her own lack of musical ability, but that she had liked to dance. I apologized that we were not smart enough yet to straighten out her limbs, but explained that some places were now using Botox with some success. "That's very interesting," she said attentively, clearly taking in every word. "Thank you very much for visiting," she added as I got up to leave. I had just been given another unexpected gift: a brief but powerful look into another person's alone and invisible world.

As the resident population at the nursing home has become dramatically more complex and more fragile, the revolving door to the hospital goes faster to give IV therapies, to evaluate any early cardiac, respiratory, or neurological symptoms, and then administer more aggressive interventional care. This sequence has become commonplace: the standard of care.

We have opened a Pandora's box where the medical care is so extensive and so quickly implemented, that many residents now live five to ten years in such an environment. Such residential care translates into a $1-million expenditure per person, not including hospital charges. At the same time, these institutions are increasingly ignoring the whole person partly because there are not enough resources and partly because it is not a high priority. Individual residents have lost most of the meaning and the value of getting up every morning. They are completely dependent on the thinly stretched staff for nearly all of their human contact. Sedentary residents are seated in the hallways around the staff as they chart their care on the flow sheets and dispense and record the medications from the rolling medication cart. If we were to make the residential-care environment fundamentally more livable, longer life there for our elders could be very desirable. If we continue our current institutional focus, long-term survival there for our elders is merely existing.

Using the Maine Approach, many more aging men and women can live in more personal settings at a lower cost. But a nursing home will still be required to manage the care of some elders. This is especially true for those with advanced dementia and extensive strokes, when they are completely incapable of any degree of independent living. Yet even this tiny minority of older individuals deserve a new paradigm. Fortunately, completely dependent, nonparticipating elders in any facility should be the exception and not the rule. In fact, most elders can live in an ordinary residential setting or in their own homes quite safely and quite successfully. We need to stop assuming otherwise and start the transformation back to a successful aging model that emphasizes community and human interaction and deemphasizes the institution and government regulation disguised as protection.

In the cases of the assisted-living facility and the nursing facility, the villain is not necessarily the facility itself, and certainly not the dedicated staff members at all levels that devote their lives to the residents assigned to them. Rather, "the enemy is us," as the Sunday comics character Pogo once famously said.

It is that we as a culture have lost touch with our elders. In an effort to provide them quality medical care, we can't see the forest for the trees. We have overlooked what this misplaced emphasis on medical care has done to the rest of the environment.

The residents of these facilities and all our elders deserve much better. The elders I have encountered and cared for at the Lincoln Home, at Cove's Edge Nursing Home, at the Schooner Cove Retirement Community, and in the Full Circle Family Medicine office have often been full of delightful surprises. They all have unique stories, hidden talents, and rich lives that few of us in the medical world were aware of. It is long past time that we reinvigorate the residential-care culture to champion their cause.

six

Forgive Me, Elsie

POETRY COMMITTED TO MEMORY IS a forgotten part of the formal education experienced by many of our elders. A couple of years ago, Rebecca, at 104, and Elsie, at 101, were both recuperating at Cove's Edge Skilled Unit after broken hips. Rebecca was living quite independently near her daughter's bed and breakfast when she fell. Elsie was struggling a bit more to live on her own in Round Pond Village with her daughter Ann living nearby. At the end of each office visit, Elsie would negotiate her next visit. If I requested a recheck in two months, she would say "four." If I suggested six months, she would say "a year." Her words regularly reminded me that she was in charge. I believe this attitude contributed in an important way to her successful aging.

One morning during their rehab stay, the nursing staff caught the two centenarian roommates dueling each other with poetry verses remembered from childhood: "The Charge of the Light Brigade" and "The Midnight Ride of Paul Revere." Their friendly competition was a testament to a bygone era and an educational approach of long ago, illustrating the power of long-term memory and offering keys to opening doors of elder engagement no one knew existed.

From my earliest days in Damariscotta, many older individuals have expressed dissatisfaction with "being put out to pasture" or being "good for nothing" or just taking up space. That poetry challenge reminded me of a poem often quoted by another memorable elder patient of mine, Nancy. A lively 90-year-old, she would refer to herself as a "one-horse shay" with all body parts disintegrating simultaneously. In a broader sense, Oliver Wendell Holmes's poem she remembered is a lesson to all of us who think we have the answers. To me it has come to represent the aspirations of this generation that generally wishes to remain useful right up until the last day of one's life. Here is a shortened version of the poem:

The Deacon's Masterpiece
Or The Wonderful "One-Hoss Shay"
A Logical Story by Oliver Wendell Holmes
(1809–1894)

Have you heard of the wonderful one-hoss shay,
That was built in such a logical way
It ran a hundred years to a day,
And then of a sudden it—ah, but stay,
I'll tell you what happened without delay,
Scaring the parson into fits,
Frightening people out of their wits,—
Have you ever heard of that, I say? . . .

. . . .

Now in building of chaises, I tell you what,
There is always *somewhere* a weakest spot,—
In hub, tire, felloe, in spring or thill,
In panel or crossbar, or floor, or sill,
In screw, bolt, throughbrace,—lurking still,
Find it somewhere you must and will,—
Above or below, or within or without,—
And that's the reason, beyond a doubt,
That a chaise *breaks down*, but doesn't *wear out*.

. . . .

So the Deacon inquired of the village folk
Where he could find the strongest oak,
That couldn't be split nor bent nor broke,—
That was for spokes and floor and sills;
He sent for lancewood to make the thills;
The crossbars were ash, from the straightest trees;
The panels of whitewood, that cuts like cheese,
But lasts like iron for things like these; . . . .

. . . .

Do! I tell you, I rather guess
She was a wonder, and nothing less!
Colts grew horses, beards turned gray,
Deacon and deaconess dropped away,
Children and grandchildren—where were they?
But there stood the stout old one-hoss shay
As fresh as on Lisbon-earthquake-day! . . .

Little of all we value here
Wakes on the morn of its hundredth year
Without both feeling and looking queer.
In fact, there's nothing that keeps its youth,
So far as I know, but a tree and truth.
(This is a moral that runs at large;
Take it.—You're welcome.—No extra charge.)

. . . .

. . .—What do you think the parson found,
When he got up and stared around?
The poor old chaise in a heap or mound,
As if it had been to the mill and ground!
You see, of course, if you're not a dunce,

How it went to pieces all at once,—
All at once, and nothing first,—
Just as bubbles do when they burst.

End of the wonderful one-hoss shay.
Logic is logic. That's all I say.

When Nancy first genuinely complained about not being able to do yoga headstands anymore, or reminisced about days when she served on the Newcastle school board, I did not comprehend how deeply felt were those losses. To her, and slowly to me, the one-horse shay analogy has come to represent not just the litany of personal health problems one can accumulate as one ages, but also, more importantly, how these problems often limit one's ability to continue to feel useful and engaged in living. She and another retirement community neighbor, Joan, would regularly commiserate about how hard it was to find good dinner table conversation in the retirement-home dining room that was not about "organ recitals" (as in heart, lung, and so on). They both wanted so much more. They wanted to avoid that exhaustive focus on specialist appointments and medical problems. They yearned to have back more of the intergenerational connections, more community service, more of the laughter and fun of earlier days. To such dreams we should all say, "Why not?"

Back in the Skilled Rehabilitation Unit, Rebecca and Elsie spurred each other on. Rather than signaling impending death, their broken hips brought unique camaraderie. The most resourceful therapists incorporated Rebecca and Elsie's shared experiences and friendly competition into their rehabilitation program. There were many more unexpected smiles that month. Rebecca returned home, coaxed forward by her irrepressible daughter. She continues to use medical care sparingly, putting more faith in independence and everyday living. She grabs what she can of each new day, living in the moment without unrealistic expectations.

Sadly, Elsie did not go home again. She moved down the corridor to the long-term-care nursing unit. Initially, she stayed in her chair, and would not participate in any more physical therapy. For some time, she could still be coaxed into recounting tales of the neighborhood she grew up in, the houses her father built, and an enormous amount of detail about people and places of a whole century. Yet she stubbornly clung to her wish to go home. Given her balance difficulties, her urinary incontinence, and her overall frailty, that choice was unavailable to her. The tears that she shed in my presence when I refused her wish to go home continue to haunt me.

It was instructive to see that sharp mind fade, and that strong will broken. She deteriorated more rapidly despite attentive care from family and staff. Although her hip had healed, we had broken her heart. I hope she can forgive me.

From the vantage point of current scientific and medical teaching, although we may not be able to extend life expectancy much beyond one hundred, we can certainly improve chronic disease management as most of us live longer.

Addressing dementia and lesser degrees of memory impairment will be paramount if we are going to effectively manage this gray tsunami. Fortunately, brain fitness is the new frontier of neuroscience. Hundreds of clinical studies worldwide now show that brain-fitness programs produce long-term improvement in memory, response time, concentration, and problem solving. Research also reveals that the brain has plasticity—that is, it can create new circuits to replace or operate alongside old circuits. It retains this ability until the day we die. We are on the threshold of finding specific brain exercises that can fine-tune specific deficits. It appears to be essential to add new content to our brain's warehouse of knowledge. Reading books, taking a class, learning a new dance, or adopting brain aerobics can begin to burn new circuits.[1] So incorporating brain fitness into a new elder paradigm is going to be increasingly important. The technological interfaces we will talk about in later chapters will lend themselves nicely to such tasks.

Equally important, we must adapt societal, family, and personal attitudes in such a way as to make this life journey rewarding to the very end. It is of no value to live twenty- or thirty-plus years beyond retirement and mostly just exist or worse yet, be waiting to die. To have nothing better to offer our elders is nothing short of a slow form of torture. We can accept what Holmes called "a general form of mild decay," but overall, we must have life be as vibrant and meaningful as possible until we die of old age. What gives life meaning must be defined by each individual, not by their caregivers.

The elders of my community regularly impress me with their insights, their humor, and most of all, the breadth and diversity of their experiences. Although it may take them longer to do something than it used to, I have been struck by how many elders are very capable of participating in their community in a meaningful way. In addition, most desire to do something for someone else. It naturally follows that if we delegate duties appropriately, most can do quite remarkable things for others. Elders are not a burden to be warehoused. The ultimate objective is not to see how long we can live but how richly we can enjoy and share that life with the world and people around us. There is a difference between surviving and living, and the sooner we willingly embrace that simple truth the fewer hearts will be broken.

The parson in "The One-Hoss Shay" provides some guidelines for a template for successful aging. Prepare early on to live a long life. Expect to be busy and useful right up until the very end of one's life. If we as a community approached this whole aging phenomenon differently, we would get a vastly different result. As the oft-heard saying goes, "If I'd known I was going to live this long, I would have taken better care of myself." Or perhaps we should paraphrase it: "If we as a community had known so many would live so long, we'd have built a better system." It is not too late to do so.

• seven •

A Better Way, We Thought

LIKE SO MANY IN THE 1990S, I thought the answers to our eldercare dilemmas lay in creating a more family-style group-home environment. The problem with institutional facilities, we theorized, was that they were too much like a hospital and too little like living at home. All we needed to do was tweak the system a bit.

So in 1995 I cofounded a nonprofit organization called the ElderCare Network. This organization grew out of a community seminar hosted by the Second Congregational Church in Newcastle and put together by the descendants of those same women's clubs that had founded the Lincoln Home. I was one of the featured speakers. Several brainstorming sessions later, a few of us called a public meeting at the Mobius Community Center in Damariscotta, and out of those enthusiastic attendees came our incorporating leadership.

Our mission was to expand options for local elders, to create alternatives to nursing homes for the increasingly frail, especially those with limited means. We recruited a diverse, hard-working board, and with the help of the Genesis Loan Fund, successfully won the Maine Department of Human Services' approval to build a noninstitutional, homelike assisted-living facility. After a two-year process of finding suitable real estate, obtaining financing through Maine State Housing Authority, Federal Home Loan Bank, Maine Women's Fund, Maine Community Development Fund, and local banks, and working with architects and contractors, hiring staff, and recruiting residents, ElderCare Network opened its doors to sixteen excited residents at Hodgdon Green in Damariscotta in the spring of 1998.

Watching the initial residents follow the building process, and seeing their excitement on moving day, matched the enthusiasm I witnessed watching my college-aged boys move into their dorms at about that same time. The incoming elder residents were fully engaged in the decisions affecting their lives and the upcoming move. This energy was in stark contrast to the usual norm preceding residential-care placement, where elders are confronted by their children and doctors at the time of a crisis that has hospitalized them. They are then suddenly told that they can no longer return home.

Twelve years later, what began with a pledged CD as collateral has grown into an assisted-living network providing housing for sixty residents, many well over 90 years old, in seven small homes located in villages throughout Lincoln County, employing forty people with a $1.8 million annual operating budget and real estate valued at $5 million. We have confounded skeptics by breaking even financially while focusing our care on the county's neediest elders.

ElderCare Network has gained statewide recognition for its unique care model and local acclaim from families and community for the pleasant, intimate atmosphere these homes provide. Most importantly, the comfort, joy, and camaraderie of each elder in this environment demonstrates the value of this approach. The social interaction is in sharp contrast to the typical institutional, residential-care-facility setting.

To give you some of the flavor of this homelike approach, I invite you to come along with me on a visit I made to these homes a couple of years ago. On May 20, 2008, along with a new board member, Samuel, I had the opportunity to visit all seven ElderCare homes in the same afternoon for a networkwide open house. They truly did embody "homelike" assisted living. The warmth and uniqueness of each home was evident upon setting foot on the premises. The highlights, appropriately enough, were the visits with residents and staff.

Our first stop was Hodgdon Green where volunteer superstars Margaret and husband Stan were taking a break at the backyard picnic table after readying the downstairs for visitors. Several residents were finishing their lunches in the dining room. Gayle and her staff were going about their business of daily care, not seeming harried by the extra tasks of the open house preparations. On the porch, Samuel engaged a couple of residents who enthusiastically expressed how fortunate they were to call this place home.

The side porch where Samuel spoke with the residents set the tone for the home. A gently sloping handicapped-accessible ramp led to this old-fashioned, large, and welcoming farmer's porch that featured wicker rocking chairs usually occupied by three or four residents enjoying the scenery. The ramp was a reminder to me of the many regulatory difficulties we overcame to start this home, our first assisted-living location. It required battling with the Maine Historic Preservation Commission over adding such a visible modification to a downtown village home.

Our intent had been to locate elders in the downtown where they could be a part of the community, walking to events when able, and within easy reach of visitors to encourage them to stop in more frequently. We also wanted the challenges of this age group to be visible and embraced by the community at large. All the preservation commission saw was a modification to a building in the designated historic district of the town. They had wanted us to locate the ramp at the back of the home, and make the handicapped residents and visitors enter from the basement via an elevator. Talk about second-class citizens! A compromise was reached before we brought adverse publicity to their hollow argument.

Next, we arrived at Wiscasset Green to find resident Jane in a stylish hat and sunglasses sunning herself independently in her wheelchair in the backyard while doubling as a greeter. Being wheelchair bound was not going to slow down this nearly ninety-year-old. Assistant manager Marge was finishing food preparations while manager Pam was running between Edgecomb and Wiscasset home responsibilities. We revisited the two upstairs rooms that could be added to the network if a rules change allowed it. Both were private, bright, spacious, and unique with full baths, but they required using the stairs. Even though the previous owner had installed a personal elevator that served him well for a decade, that same elevator had been declared unusable by our state inspectors because it did not conform to commercial code. As a result, two valuable elder rooms have remained vacant for most of the last several years.

A few residents were in their rooms, with television-program background noise begging for a few more volunteers to provide other activity. We even got a chance to respond to some of resident Barbara's medical concerns, hopefully saving her a doctor's-office visit. Board member and RN Ruth was there to field follow-up questions. First-time visitor and architect Bill arrived to get some pointers on how we manage the network as he contemplated starting an elder home himself.

Edgecomb Green was our next stop. Board member Bob and staff member Crystal were there to greet us. We checked out the back porch to see what improvements would allow renewed access to that important feature. Getting outside, being right in the trees, surveying the woods, feeling the breeze, listening to the birds are such important connections to the natural world for these residents. Yet the state building inspector was quick to make that entire deck off-limits when one narrow plank showed signs of excess wear.

A similar regulatory issue here was the ongoing battle over the massive commercial-range hood—installed per regulations—that dwarfs the galley kitchen, sucks all of the heat out of the downstairs, prevents residents from lingering at the dining room table after meals for conversation, and has even allowed food left out on the counter overnight to freeze! When will we ever learn?

Of course, the staff were all super, representing the welcoming and caring attitude we all prize. Resident Connie graciously showed us her room upstairs as we marveled at how the room's dormer and skylight created a one-of-a-kind home for her. She loved it.

We then drove down to Boothbay Green where manager Elizabeth and two staff members, Angie and Jean, proudly offered a delicious variety of cookies all made by the residents themselves. They told us of their upcoming garden plans, organized by two other residents who are accomplished gardeners.

Board member Tom added to the welcoming atmosphere. We were impressed with the whole feel of the home: a bright, airy kitchen and eating area, and an old-fashioned, wainscoted living room. The den was graced with dark-stained French doors—but their survival was threatened by the fire marshal declaring them not up to the code requiring solid-core doors next to hallway stairs. What a shame to lose this historic feature and its connection to a front hall with a stained glass window and a curved, gracious banister because of a bureaucratic detail. This home surely served a six-member family well for many decades before we asked it to serve six elder residents. It continued to be an ongoing battle to get regulators to think of elders and their lives in noninstitutional terms.

Around the corner in a cozy newer wing, we met Clifton happily resting with and feeding the resident three-legged house cat from the shelter. As he shared his health and fishing stories, and stroked the sleeping cat, it was hard to tell who was happier with the accommodations. Across the hall, we were greeted by Katherine, the daughter of George Washington and his wife Martha (honest!), as she proudly showed us her family portraits and urged us to look around *her* lovely home and visit her again whenever we wished.

Next, we drove around the peninsula to get to Round Pond Green, where an expansive front porch and the most elaborate buffet greeted us. Board member Martha and longtime supporters of ElderCare Network Joyce and Bob made us feel right at home as did residents Ruby, Jane, and Delores. Each again reiterated how lucky they felt to have found such a special home, although Ruby commented she would love to be back in her own home in Nobleboro. Since she had worked almost full-time as a hostess at local restaurants until she was ninety, I would not have expected any different remark from her.

A couple of employees engaged us in a very spirited discussion about their challenges trying to get by on their current wages while raising families, buying food and putting gas in the car. They were effusive about their love of the residents, their work, and the home in general but opened our eyes to the reality of what our dedicated staff do for only $9.00 per hour. I explained the board's frustration with the financial realities of having the state as effectively our only source of revenue. They volunteered to go with us to lobby for needed changes, and I suggested we find a way to take them up on their offer. They put a very compelling face on the issues we have raised to our state legislators.

I had a lot to ponder as I drove to Waldoboro Green where the biggest party of the day was going on. The dining room was full of staff, residents, and volunteers talking, laughing, and eating. The ball field behind the house was in full swing, and school kids passed by the front walk on their way home from the Miller School. That was the main attraction for our board in choosing that location: visible from the elementary school, town ball field, VFW hall, and in sight of a bucolic brook. It was our goal to locate elders in the middle of things in their communities.

Resident Barbara, newly home from the hospital and a Cove's Edge rehab stay, enthusiastically took us on a guided tour of every inch of Waldoboro Green. She also introduced us to all the other residents, including Midell and Rowena. Rowena delighted us with her artwork, note cards, and entrepreneurial spirit. She had installed her own photocopier in her room so that she could produce more note cards for sale at lower cost. Board member Beth and manager Kim rounded out the appeal of this special home. It is our only radiant-heated, passive solar home, proving one can provide affordable comfort for elder residents in a green building.

I finally arrived at Jefferson Green in late afternoon. The staff, including manager Joyce, had prepared the dining room with lots of goodies. One resident, Jeanette, gave us an animated tour made more memorable by her expressive language difficulties made worse when she got excited. And she was excited! Two other residents on the couch in the living room, Beulah and Dot, proudly recounted the story of the arrival of the carved folk art owl on the hearth that they had found at the dump. They all made us feel right at home. Another member of the community we met used the open house as an opportunity to become a regular volunteer there.

When we returned to Hodgdon Green we caught up again with staff, residents, and volunteers all unwinding together after a very successful day. We were impressed with the camaraderie among all, the gentle teasing, the very natural blending of all ages and status and reason for being there. It absolutely felt like a big family party and was as far removed from anything institutional as all of us could hope. We all felt rightfully proud of seeing the vision we shared ten years ago become such a remarkable reality.

The day had been a celebration of the possible, one that absolutely reaffirmed why we were doing everything we could to keep ElderCare Network alive and well. So many had played important roles in its success.

That happy day was three years ago. It seems so much longer than that. Despite the festivities of our tour, the financial picture of the ElderCare Network was bleak and deteriorating further. As I write this book, the future of these seven wonderful homes is in doubt. The reasons for this uncertainty are not difficult to discern.

Over the last decade, larger upscale assisted-living complexes have been developed, attracting most of the community's private-pay residents. ElderCare Network remained the only Lincoln County option for elders on state assistance. It has become routine for the private-pay assisted-living facilities to evict residents once their money has run out. Our modest operation has thus become a refuge of last resort for those totally dependent upon state-funded care. Our payer mix went from 67 percent to 90 percent state-assistance residents. To make matters worse, the state also implemented a complex case-mix formula from the nursing home world, and the budget steadily tightened.

Then came years of skyrocketing energy costs on top of steadily rising food, labor, and insurance expenses. With state reimbursement increasing only 1.9 percent in five years, ElderCare Network is tottering on the brink of financial insolvency. Despite uniform sympathy from legislators and regulators for years, the equation has not changed. State coffers are empty too. Additional stopgap measures were pursued. We were able to refinance loans, and we invested in weatherization projects using hard-won grant money. Every other cost-containment efficiency has been adopted. It is uncertain whether that will be enough.

Despite our better-way vision and execution with seven wonderful homes, the fundamental issue remains. Neither ElderCare Network nor any other entity can provide the requisite eldercare at a low enough cost. The state of Maine was paying us $2,390 per resident per month when the private-pay facilities in our town were charging their residents $5,000 to $6,200 for a comparable level of care. Meanwhile, these private-pay competitors cherry-pick the well-off, and cavalierly kick them into the street when they can no longer afford to pay. They end up on ElderCare Network's doorstep or occasionally are transferred to the nursing home with a rare open bed. In our community, Fieldcrest Manor Nursing Home closed with very little warning when a national nursing home corporation bought the property and decided too many residents there were on state assistance. Families scrambled to find places for these unfortunate long-term-care residents.

ElderCare Network was doing a phenomenal job at a bargain price, and still the state could not afford it. It did not matter how efficiently we were run. It did not matter that ElderCare Network was blazing an important new trail creating small, noninstitutional homes. We needed to go further. Being solely reliant on the government of Maine and its taxpayers had proven to be unsustainable. In the long run, we needed to find new sources of revenue or we would fail. An essential service would disappear. You would think the government would appreciate that fact and work with us to survive. Think again.

eight

Government Regulation
beyond Reason

DESPITE THE ONGOING FINANCIAL challenges of providing homelike top-quality assisted living, the most difficult part over the years at ElderCare Network has been the almost adversarial relationship with our supposed partners in state government. There is a widespread attitude that our approach, and definitely our execution, as a provider would be substandard without their vigilant oversight.

Shortly after ElderCare Network was formed, we filed our application for Hodgdon Green in response to the Maine Department of Health and Human Services' "request for proposals." When our application was the highest ranked proposal in the state, we expected a collaborative relationship with the various agencies in that department to help us get our doors open.

It was anything but. Every agency seemed to have a political agenda. Each treated us as ignorant supplicants lucky to have its attention. Now, maybe if this was the late 1950s with scandals rocking the industry, one could understand the attitude. But this was something else altogether.

So, after navigating the entire process, getting our final approvals, and having opened our doors, we got the attention of then Maine governor Angus King, who arranged a meeting in his office with our board leadership to elicit feedback from us about the process. We came prepared to outline the obstacles other communities would face if they were to follow our lead. Mind you, we needed nothing further from state government at that point. We were only there to help the next guy learn from our experience. And the governor himself had specifically recruited a new commissioner for the Department of Health and Human Services to promote progressive elder residential care statewide. So we expected a receptive audience.

If there were a prize for cluelessness when it comes to politics it would be sitting on my mantel.

Governor King assembled many of the agency heads to sit in on our conversation. So we talked and vented about the process. Since it was a private meeting without any press, I figured that the participants could handle our attempt at constructive criticism. The icy reception we suffered there took two years to thaw.

Among our criticisms, still valid today, was the fact that the Maine funding authority, which existed to help fill the gap to finance projects such as ours, was more risk averse than the local banks we were working with. Despite only being asked to guarantee half of the funding, the pile of required paperwork was absurd. The local bank's dossier was tiny by comparison. Even today, with national interest rates at historic lows, we have 8.5 percent loans with the Maine State Housing Authority that they will not renegotiate. If we could just pay market-rate interest, the available cash could go immediately toward other expenses. But the ongoing relationship remains inflexible, and the lender that was supposed to be part of the solution has become a serious part of the problem.

Our battle with the Maine Historic Preservation Commission over how to modify an existing downtown structure to accommodate handicapped elders without altering the architectural lines of the building was another clear example of the left hand not knowing what the right hand was doing or more exactly "wanted to do."

We met obstacles from other government agencies too. The fire marshal's office from the beginning was obstructionist, dictatorial, and seemed to act autonomously from other parts of state government. The sprinkler system that was mandated for our homelike assisted-living facility of sixteen residents, which was literally across the street from the fire department, required installation of a new six-inch-diameter water line from the main in the street. I suspect that if we ever used it, the rest of the town's water would slow to a trickle. The massive, shiny cast-iron valve system in our dirt-floor partial basement looks more robust and elaborate than that at Damariscotta Mills, a local hydroelectric plant. The cost was enough to eliminate some of our preferred building amenities.

Another fire marshal bone of contention was door swings and door closers. Our downstairs resident bathroom shower-room door was designed by our architect to open inward so as to not interfere with resident traffic from the main hall and stairwell to the main dining room. This design was disallowed because of fire marshal concerns. For the decade since, frail first-floor residents with their walkers and wheelchairs have to navigate around this large, heavy, outward-opening doorway. Every day it causes problems.

On the second floor, a spry 100-year-old resident has multiple bruises covering both forearms because heavy spring-loaded door closers were required on all doorways opening on the hall where the stairs are located. She must negotiate two of these to get from the elevator to her bedroom. Only because of her cautious perseverance does she get into and out of her room without assistance and without being knocked over. Our bureaucrats are fooling themselves to think they are protecting her.

The state building inspector also places our residents in peril. This office regularly inspects to see that the water temperature at the sinks in bathrooms and kitchen is 135 degrees to reduce infection risk. Scalded resident skin is of no concern. In an assisted-living home where the goal is to encourage independence and privacy, and where the average age at times approaches 90 years old, it is illogical and downright dangerous not to turn down these water temperatures. Our dishwashers have a commercial temperature booster and sterilization cycles that function independently from this water supply, so a public-health argument was not valid. But in the "check the box" mentality of the state inspector the big picture was irrelevant.

But the finance authority, fire marshal, and state inspector were, by comparison, all lightweights. The Maine Licensing Division was our biggest adversary. From the beginning, even resident room-size restrictions were unreasonable. The Maine regulations appropriately have minimum room sizes for those receiving state assistance, but also having maximum size restrictions troubled us. We were building a new wing and were not allowed to build a resident bedroom larger than 120 square feet. How could we logically expect an elder to willingly and cheerfully move from her own home or apartment to such a small room? We were trying to create homelike, welcoming residential space that would overcome elders' resistance to get the help they needed. We were being stymied at literally every turn. We ended up creating an entry foyer in each room with an oversized almost walk-in closet to provide a little more space without violating size regulations.

Also we were not allowed to use state funding for a residents' activity room or for additional small-group sitting or visiting spaces outside of their own bedrooms. So we enlarged hallways and corridors by an extra foot, put a window and chair at the end of the hall, and did not call it a sitting room. We needed to creatively work around the restrictions to provide the space to make the home more appealing. We then needed to seek private funds to offer additional common space.

The next issue with the licensing and building division was that of call bells. Historically, there have been pull chains or emergency call buttons in bathrooms or next to beds, for use in high-fall-risk areas. We preferred to offer more modern personal emergency-response buttons that the resident could wear, and would be usable wherever they had a problem and not just in predesignated places. No dice. We could put in both systems but were required to hard-wire the walls. I even submitted a personal survey from nursing home head nurses representing a cumulative 150 years of long-term care experience that vouched that no one among them had ever seen a resident use a hardwired emergency cord. Still to no avail. So no innovation and no application of common sense.

The next regulatory issue was much more serious. All low-income residents on state assistance are required to turn over all but $70 per month of their Social Security check as well as all other income to the state to be eligible for funded residential care. Out of this $70 per month, residents must pay for their telephone and cable or Internet in their rooms, as these services are not deemed a reimbursable expense for ElderCare Network to pay for them. As more and more Medicare and Medicaid drug plans do not cover any over-the-counter medications, these residents are also expected to cover the costs of their aspirin, calcium, and vitamin D, iron and multivitamins, as well as stomach-acid suppressant medications, Tylenol, bowel medications, and more out of their own pockets. All on $70 a month.

So how can this proud cohort even pay for other near essentials like toiletries, a haircut, an article of clothing, or, God forbid, a movie, an ice cream, or a birthday card for a grandchild? This is beyond outrageous. We are demanding these elders forgo basics that the rest of us would not stand for. Their only fault is that often they have lived long enough to outlast their savings.

The building restrictions, the inspection issues, and the fiscal stinginess pale in comparison to what the resident-assessment process says and does about the human interactions between staff and individuals in the eldercare homes. It is difficult to calmly address the cost in time and staff hours that results from this bureaucratic regulation as everyone's efforts are spent complying with rules that rarely impact the quality of a resident's life.

I do not believe that many people I have met in state government like this situation any more than I do. It is critical that the environment fostered in residential-care facilities truly addresses and responds to the diverse needs of its residents. To produce a comprehensive solution will require broad collaboration and leadership from many state agencies. It will also require innovation and courage. The intent of many regulations was to protect residents from substandard conditions. In practice, many of these rules and the manner in which they are enforced actually harm residents, imperil the financial survival of the places in which they live, and do nothing to enrich their lives. A brighter future for many elders' lives rests on our abilities to shape a new paradigm together.

• nine •

The State of Maine vs. Common Sense

THE GRAVEST AFFRONT TO OUR ELDERS in assisted-living facilities derives from the current licensing and payment rules for those receiving government assistance. Those rules allocate care based on a medical model, and that model is taken from the nursing home world—not the world elders inhabit in assisted living. Not only does this mean that their real needs may go unaddressed, but it also means their caregivers' time is often spent on elaborate, sometimes useless paperwork rather than on their care. And it can also mean that the facilities where these elders live can be jeopardized by a few wrong answers on a multiple-choice questionnaire. We learned this the hard way.

Granted, the big, broad, assisted-living world covers a vast expanse of individuals, from those who are just a small step away from being able to live independently at home to those who require extensive assistance for nearly all daily activities but still don't require the intensive individual care offered at a nursing home.

To qualify for state funding, assisted-living residents must need help with a certain number of activities of daily living (or ADLs). Their caregivers must use assessment forms called minimum data sets (MDS) to tally their capabilities. The scores from these assessments determine their reimbursement. Additionally, the assisted-living facilities themselves must now follow rules developed for the traditionally more regulated nursing home world to get licensed. And these rules are enforced aggressively.

In 2006, Hodgdon Green, ElderCare's flagship homelike assisted-living residence, was fined by the state of Maine for allegedly inappropriately completing such MDS forms. We continued to appeal the penalty, and at long last the state of Maine hearing officer finally granted us an administrative hearing in April 2009 to contest the sanctions levied against ElderCare Network. The story of that legal struggle shows the ugliest side of highly regulated assisted living.

When I arrived at the hearing with our executive director, business manager, and nursing coordinator, the hearing officer notified us of the rules of the hearing. Lacking formal legal representation, one of us would be designated our legal counsel. Both sides would be allowed to call witnesses and to cross-examine the other side's witnesses. Opening and closing statements would be entered into the record. The entire proceeding would be taped, and the hearing officer would issue his verdict within a few weeks of the hearing.

With that introduction, as surreal as it seemed to me, a full-fledged trial was on. I had come prepared to answer questions, not deliver an opening argument. All I had was a written summary. I also was not expecting the state's assistant attorney general to be my opponent. This was a much higher profile case than I expected.

The $8,000 fine imposed upon us by the state of Maine may have been small change to a large nursing home corporation; but that kind of fine could drive a bus over our struggling operation.

I gave our appeal my best shot in the hope that common sense might prevail against all odds. What follows is part of the written documents supplied to the hearing officer. I apologize for how complicated the scoring system is, and therefore how tedious is my explanation of the stated deficiencies. Unfortunately, that detail reflects our current payment system for homelike assisted living. No home trying hard to care for our elders should have to stoop so low. Here is what I said.

> I have been a family physician in Damariscotta for over twenty years. I am board certified in family medicine

with an additional certificate in geriatrics. I have also served as the medical director of Cove's Edge Nursing Home and the Lincoln Home Assisted-Living Facility. Twelve years ago, I cofounded a nonprofit organization, ElderCare Network, to address the residential needs of Lincoln County's frail, low-income elders. Today, we remain the sole assisted-living provider for elders on state assistance, housing sixty elders, most over ninety years old and more than 90 percent dependent on MaineCare (state financial assistance).

I continue to serve as the president of the ECN board working diligently to provide compassionate home-like care while we try to make ends meet in difficult economic times. We have received less than a 1 percent cumulative rate increase in six years, while in just the last three years our costs are up 25 percent overall. Some energy line items are up over 200 percent. We continue to receive statewide and community praise for our work.

Needless to say, the sanctions we received in mid-2008 for issues cited in December 2006 and July 2007 hit us particularly hard both professionally and financially. Such sanctions suggest that we billed inappropriately for care we did not deliver, overcharging the state, and insinuate that we engaged in unsafe practices in our homes. We investigated the allegations and disagree with the methods and the conclusions.

Over the years right up to the present, our auditors and cost preparers, and the reviewers at the Bureau of Elder and Adult Services have consistently made comments about how low our "case-mix index" was. Compared to other assisted-living facilities, despite housing some very frail residents for more than a decade of progressive aging in place, our daily payment rate was still very low. They have questioned how we could survive on such low reimbursement. In fact, we are struggling, and a $10,000 fine could put another nail in our coffin.

With that as background, I would like to take apart the "errors" that led to the sanctions. In July 2007, *five* resident charts were subjected to a focused review. *Three* errors in coding were found, leading to a 60 percent error-rate calculation, according to the state's formula. For that percentage error rate, department regulation required Hodgdon Green to return *10 percent of total revenue* received from the state during the entire preceding six months. These are very high stakes. Moreover, I believe the errors are statistically insignificant and substantively unimportant. The outcome of such an action threatens the survival of a valuable community resource for sixty elders.

I have reviewed the Residential Care Assessment form in some detail, and, excluding the demographic data, tallied about 415 statements about each resident's mental and physical health that our nurse coordinator must score every six months. Using this new denominator, as I argue you should, the error rate is about 0.001 percent, that is, three errors out of 2,730 statements, not 60 percent as the state has alleged.

Now for the specific errors.

Error no. 1. Betty is a 100-year-old, twelve-year-long resident of Hodgdon Green currently under hospice care due to her fragile overall health. In section G of her MDS form, the scorer is asked to assess that she "needs help with set up" either preparing for meals or for washing up, and the choices are 0, 1, or 2, with 0 signifying being "completely independent," i.e., does it all by herself; 2 means "needs help all the time," and

1 represents "needs some help and/or supervision." It was this middle category that was checked. Our staff and board stand by that scoring as consistent with the care delivered for that resident in question at that time. However, the documentation required to substantiate selecting that choice is lacking. The scorer must find three episodes recorded in the aides' notes during the fourteen-day look-back period that specifically mention that service being delivered. The reviewer did find three notations, but two of these were on the same day and therefore one was disallowed. Now mind you, our scorer is the clinical-care coordinator for Hodgdon Green, and in our small home often assists the aides in providing regular care to this and all our sixteen residents. She knows them all exceptionally well. And, in this instance, to an outside reviewer like me, I believe she picked the only appropriate choice, i.e., "some of the time."

Error no. 2. Marjorie was a 96-year-old, sweet, moderately demented resident who recently broke her hip and subsequently expired postoperatively from a heart attack at Mercy Hospital in Portland. In section E of her MDS form for the time period in question, she was scored as having "a sad mood" "some of the time" with the choices in this category again being 0, 1, and 2 for "never," "some of the time," or "all of the time." The requirement in *this* section is that you find up to three notations in seven days or four times in thirty days to support the "some of the time" choice. The reviewer only found three notations in nine days that month and again tagged that entire chart with its other 415 MDS inquiries as being in error. Again, a violation of a strict interpretation of the coding rules but hardly a serious offense. As her treating physician for her depression during the period in question, I contend that 1 was an appropriate tally for this statement; and suspect she was actually an under-coded as a 2. Certainly, there was no fraudulent attempt on anyone's part to garner reimbursement we were not entitled to receive.

Error no. 3. Elsie is a 95-year-old legally blind woman with one of our highest case-mix indexes of 1.37. In the MDS category for "special treatments," the scorer is asked to list the number of new physician orders during a two-week look-back period. In this instance, the two-week look-back was September 1 to September 15. Unfortunately for us, her birthday was September 7. When the coder read the date of her birthday as the date of the orders, she mistakenly gave her a score of 5. [She was counted as having 5 new physician orders in early September rather than noticing that all her order sheets had her date of birth on them!] This was an inadvertent human misreading. In reality, in an average month, this high-needs resident does have frequent order changes, and does require a high level of care. So I sincerely doubt that the result affected our reimbursement. Ironically, at other times, state reviewers had indeed offered comments to our scorer that we were often under-coding on the care of this resident specifically.

In the other time period during which the sanctions were levied, December 2006, *eight* charts were reviewed; *three* "errors" were found; and a 37 percent error rate assigned with the attendant required financial penalty. Again, here are the violations that were graded as "errors."

Error no. 1. Grace, a 99-year-old resident of Hodgdon Green for twelve years, is under treatment for delusional thinking. When she becomes delusional, her usual pattern is not to start talking bizarrely, but to withdraw to her room and be less interactive with residents and staff. In section J of her MDS form under "medication side effects," a yes or no answer is scored for "delusions." The scorer marked yes when the aides' notes supported the oft-repeated pattern of withdrawn behavior on the part of this resident. But no specific mention was made by the entry-level staff of the words "delusional behavior." I challenge you to find a practicing physician, let alone an entry-level nurse's aide, who is not often challenged by making such a distinction. I give our staff credit for identifying this behavior as well as they did.

Error no. 2. Elsie, in section G under "toilet use," was scored as a 3 for "extensive assistance needed" with the supporting documentation requiring three notations in a seven-day look-back period when in actuality three notations were found in nine days.

Error no. 3. Vera, in section E of her MDS form under "Mood and Behavior," scored a 1 for "some of the time" when "crying," "tearful," and "insomnia" were the allowed qualifiers, but the supporting notations were again just shy of the allowed threshold for "some of the time." I again submit that this was the only correct choice even though the documentation may have been partially lacking.

In summary, I hope you can see why we feel that the financial penalties assessed are unusually and inappropriately harsh. Moreover, I believe that the MDS forms in the individual charts in question were coded in such a way as to truthfully represent the state of the residents at the time care was assessed. The few "errors" found do not in any significant way change the status of these individuals. I do not believe they are grounds for reprimand or financial penalty. ElderCare Network does not warrant the connotation of "sanctions" for the issues outlined above. If anything, this scoring system and the penalties assessed will lead to wholesale under-coding to avoid additional sanctions and further reduce the already inadequate reimbursement system, thereby threatening the survival of those facilities that strive to provide care for our state's poorest residents.

I strongly urge those responsible for developing and enforcing this coding system to take a fresh look at the impact on residential care of the current MDS system. While providing a very thorough assessment of each individual resident, is such detail necessary and justifiable given the valuable time and resources expended at both ends of the process?

It was an Alice in Wonderland experience. The errors were trivial, but we were actually on trial for them. Somehow the state had lost its way and seemed to be proceeding on the assumption that some well-heeled residential-care developer was going to skip a jet payment and pull $8,000 from his otherwise excessive profits. Did they understand ours was a *not-for-profit* organization and ultimately it would be the patients that would be hurt?

When the state's witnesses testified, the absurdity of the situation reached a new level.

Sharon Stanley of the Division of Program Integrity, and Lillian Phillips, RN, case-mix nurse, were the principal witnesses for the state. Ms. Stanley defined her job as "safeguarding the state's MaineCare assets from waste, fraud, and abuse." However, she stated unequivocally that she saw no evidence of waste, fraud, or abuse on the part of Hodgdon Green in this matter. She further stated that she would categorize these coding "errors" as "simple human errors." Ms. Phillips stated that during her near decade-long relationship of reviewing records at Hodgdon Green, there had been no pattern of coding errors. In fact, she pointed out that we had had a zero error rate both before and after the reviews in question.

Ms. Phillips, in particular, and department inspection divisions in general, have been uniformly complimentary of the care delivered at Hodgdon Green, the homelike atmosphere they have witnessed there, and the valuable role ElderCare Network serves. At no time, during the testimony or cross-examination of any witness, was there the faintest hint that any "error" uncovered would have resulted in any harm to any resident. In no way would the coding issues have compromised the care of any resident. In fact, the counterargument could be made that coding these charts "correctly" in the instances cited would have underreported the needs of the residents in question and potentially deprived Hodgdon Green of the funds needed to serve its residents appropriately.

Despite the positive view of the two inspectors, the hearing officer ruled in favor of his department, and ElderCare Network began paying the sanctions penalty. I do not believe any rational person would conclude that these errors reflected adversely on the quality of the care delivered. To the contrary, I suspect most readers would be appalled that this is the kind of regulation governing the care of our elders. Was this truly the way the state of Maine should be investing its tax dollars?

I am sure most of the families of these residents would object to Hodgdon Green staff taking valuable time away from their caregiving duties to comply with such onerous and pointless documentation. Most would question the wisdom of such a system's priorities. Nevertheless, reliance on this inadequate scoring system continues, and new revisions to it are expected to bring even harsher penalties and stricter enforcement. The madness continues.

The aftermath of this administrative hearing also points out some of the other weaknesses in government regulations. I have had a close working relationship with Department of Health and Human Services throughout the last decade, and I have had the opportunity to meet with Commissioner Brenda Harvey several times about elder issues. She has always been a champion of progressive eldercare, and complimentary of the work we were doing in Lincoln County.

Since her name was officially on the verdict of our appeal, I wrote her to request an informal "for future reference" review of this whole sanctions chapter to help other elder residents down the road. She did not even know about the case in question. It barely crossed her desk, if at all. So despite her dedicated leadership at the top of the largest department in state government, the likelihood that she can change or even influence the culture below her is small. Commissioners are sheltered from the decisions made in their names. There is a hopeless disconnect between the policy aims of senior leadership and the execution on the ground.

Residential care has come a long way from the scandals of elder neglect and overt fraud that characterized the conditions of the poor farms, the almshouses, some of the homes for the aged, and some of the nursing homes of the 1960s and 1970s. The advent of assisted living offered the promise of a significant departure from the pitfalls of the nursing home world. But the regulatory jungle that is now the standard of care threatens elders just as profoundly by robbing their caregivers of the dollars and time that could otherwise be used to provide them care, comfort, and companionship. The current regulatory environment wastes equally valuable state resources that could be better spent promoting more enlightened policy and leadership for elder residential care.

Complaining about this state of affairs is pointless. What is needed is a means to separate the bureaucrats from the process—to create and implement a very different approach.

ten

Breakthrough: The Roots
of the Maine Approach

JUST WHAT WOULD THAT NEW approach look like? With the benefit of twenty years caring for elders in all sorts of situations, including the Lincoln Home, Cove's Edge, and the ElderCare Network, I have concluded that a unique home-care model works the best for all involved. It costs less. The patients are happier and healthier. There is a greater opportunity for neighbors and friends to become part of a support team. And the best part is that our elders are restored to their rightful place in the community.

Gradually, over the last few years, our dedicated band has tried to shape our observations into a coherent, comprehensive new elder paradigm. We have observed and interviewed many elders as we've tried to craft the kind of community support systems, opportunities for involvement, and assisted-living facilities that make sense for them. We have borrowed from many sectors. We continuously refine the shape of our model.

Over the course of all this thinking and rethinking, a few guiding principles have emerged:

- Emphasize elders living in their own homes as long as possible.
- Engage elders as fully as possible in living every day fully.
- Empower elders to take back control of their lives.
- Promote elder independence and interdependence.

- Encourage intergenerational contact and relationships.
- Offer diverse volunteer opportunities for everyone regardless of age.
- Find volunteering opportunities for even the most infirm elder.
- Offer a variety of support choices, but insist on as few as possible.
- Showcase and celebrate whenever possible elder wisdom and experience.
- Provide a reasonable level of safety and reassurance.
- Elicit and refine elder goals and new or old interests.
- Make connections to family, friends, and community.
- Harness elder talents and abilities as an untapped resource.

I've already explained that we do this by combining affordable, yet amazing, high-tech monitoring devices with a well-organized volunteer team, and a central core of trained health-care providers. But I haven't explained one crucial point: We also start from the premise that our mission is not to protect the elder from every conceivable danger but rather to let them live as much as possible.

The Maine Approach requires an appreciation of the individual. It presumes that we appreciate the diversity of our elder cohort. It insists that we tune into their goals and their aspirations. It demands that we look at our elders in an entirely new light. A regimented, institutional setting cannot meet their needs. Let me put human faces on what I mean.

Arletta

Arletta was not first-and-foremost a frail 95-year-old with end-stage renal disease who needed to be propped up at the piano by her nephew. She was a lifelong musician who started an all-girls jazz band in the 1930s in the small town of Jefferson, Maine. She still loved to play "Sweet Georgia Brown" on the piano. A couple of weeks before she died, she entertained family and friends at the keyboard with her honky-tonk repertoire. She then apologized, or more correctly pointed out, that she would have performed better if the piano had been properly tuned. She still had her musical ear.

She was the same woman who, ten years back, when I was giving her a tour of our new assisted-living home in town, coyly remarked on how she preferred the two connected rooms in the remodeled front of the building, in case she and her husband wanted to snuggle. How many residential eldercare planners take that need into account?

Ginny

Ginny is not primarily the 87-year-old with Alzheimer's disease whose hands hurt because she cannot remember to use her carpal tunnel splints. She is a former elementary school teacher who ran a restaurant with her assistant-principal husband for many years during the summers. She is also a double-headed-doll maker who still felt very comfortable surrounded by her crafts as well as her word searches. She loves to flirt and meets people easily. Clearly, this thumbnail sketch of her tells you much more about her than her medical chart. You want to interact with her and not just pass her by. She should not be stereotyped by her memory impairment.

Bobby

Bobby was not just an 84-year-old with valvular heart disease, asthma, renal insufficiency, anemia, and intermittent confusion. He was a former dairy farmer who retired to play a lot of golf. He was an unlikely member of the country-club set. He had raised a few beef critters for extra cash, and was a very close friend of the other serious farmers in the county. They collaborated and shared ideas on how to make a living farming. He also loved to attend dances and have a little too much to drink. He built himself a retirement home on the lake, and wanted to look across the fields of hay and have wildflowers by his sliding glass door. Watching the Red Sox or the PGA rounded out a perfect day for him. He had so many topics that he enjoyed talking about. Any visit with him was a treat. His home was where he wanted to be, no matter what.

Florence

Florence was more than a 93-year-old feisty woman, legally blind from her macular degeneration. She loved to tell stories about growing up on a farm. She delivered a pretty clean joke with decent timing. Florence remembered when her town of Waldoboro had a mill and a laundry that ran on water power. She could recount a typical day before widespread electricity. When prompted, she definitely came out of her shell. She performed comfortably on stage at our "Young At Heart" elder talent show in the high school cafeteria when given the opportunity. Her strained relationship with her family relegated her to far more isolation than she preferred. I suspect her poor vision hardened her attitude, making her a tougher nut to crack.

Marion

Marion is 90 and resists all my attempts to connect her with others. Her memory is sharp. Her talents are extraordinary. She received her PhD in biology at the time of Watson and Crick, and she will enthrall you with the detailed accounts of post-doctoral science fifty years ago and her fruit-fly experiments. She has turned her methodical mind to painting delicate Ukrainian eggs for the last twenty years, and focuses doggedly on getting to the next craft fair despite her increasingly limiting arthritis. Marion insists she does not like people in spite of her body language to the contrary. She also cannot believe anyone would have an interest in her personally, only in her crafts. So our conversations on these far-flung subjects needed to be spontaneous and even arranged a little deviously.

As Jerry Friedman discovered when interviewing and photographing elders for his book, *The Wisdom of Our Elders*, there are a great many secrets and treasures locked within the minds of older Americans. Most of these gems are going to stay there because the holders are either unable or unwilling to share them. Discovery requires us to be patient; something we're not very good at being. Moreover, this valuable cohort is segregated from the community at large. Few people come in contact with them on a regular basis. Most care-givers are too busy paying attention to medical needs to notice or discuss anything else.

These snapshots of a few elders begin to showcase the diversity of the elder cohort. Their lives defy being defined only by medical conditions and treatments. They deserve to be embraced for what they bring to the table. The goal of the Maine Approach is to try to do justice to their legacy by creating a model they would applaud. The take-home message is that if we look for it, there is a gem in nearly every elder encounter.

My most dramatic personal example of this realization occurred more than a decade ago. I had been assigned an evening admission to the hospital of a new patient, a woman in her nineties, with high blood pressure who was too weak to go home. After a few moments of complaining about missing another evening with my family, and while waiting for lab tests to return, I decided to make the most of the situation. I went to Ella's bedside, and started up a conversation. "Tell me what you did for work when you were younger," I began. "I was a hairdresser in Augusta," she replied matter-of-factly. "I don't know much about Augusta," I continued, "What part of the city did you live in?" "My last address there was the Blaine House." (For those not from Maine, that is the governor's mansion). "I do know where that is," I smiled. "My husband was the governor, Fred Payne, 1948." "Where did you live next?" I was all ears now. "Washington." "So he was elected to the Senate?" "Yes, he was the junior senator to Margaret Chase Smith." So began one of the most fascinating hours I have ever spent. This woman was all alone in a cubicle on a gurney. Her appearance was very ordinary. She even looked quite impoverished. She told me in great detail about Senator Joe and Mrs.

McCarthy, the Senate hearings on Un-American Activities, Dwight Eisenhower, and Margaret Chase Smith. And from her vantage point, it was more of a people's history of that Maine era, and very down-to-earth. Delightful. As usual, I was handsomely rewarded for digging a little deeper.

We need to constantly look way beyond the medical chart. Let us visit several other elders to further illustrate the key points. I want to impress you with the sheer magnitude of the cohort. I want you to identify with the fact that I am not talking about a few isolated elders. I am writing not only about a veritable gray tsunami but also about a hidden treasure trove.

Helen

At 96, Helen's needs were very simple. Yet the high-quality $10,000-per-month local nursing home could not meet them. She wanted to be in her own home, surrounded by the memories of a lifetime of family and activity. She wanted to get up when she wanted to, fix herself something to eat when she wanted to, watch the evening news when she wanted to, be in her own living room and entertain the occasional relative or friend in her own environment when she wanted to. More than two and a half years earlier, with her daughter's consent and our support, she moved back home, and was as happy as she could be, despite her incredibly fragile health, until the day she died peacefully in her own home.

Flora

Ninety-seven-year-old Flora wonders why she cannot still be home. Her favorite company was her cat. She loved watching the bold chipmunks and birds on the deck off her bedroom. She politely restricted visitors to the few who did not tire her out with incessant questions. She now sits in the nursing home doorway or self-propels her wheelchair through the hallways, asking why she cannot return home, and who is that stranger in her bedroom?

Gladys

Ninety-year-old Gladys lives next door to her attentive daughter's bed and breakfast. But her forgetfulness taxes their relationship. The demands of the business frequently take precedence over Gladys' request for a cup of tea or a game of Scrabble. She needs a companion who can deftly fill in a few gaps, someone who extends the otherwise reasonable living accommodations and spells her daughter, preferably someone who will treat her as an equal, and not act condescendingly toward her.

Adele

Adele is 78 and loves daily long walks in the neighborhood in which she grew up. Her dementia worries her daughters, but moving her to a new environment would strip her of her remaining independence. The kitchen is too cluttered, but she knows her way around it and she manages. She loves weekly visits with her childhood friend Kathryn at the local assisted-living home, the two chattering away like a couple of schoolgirls. Both have significant dementia, but their relationship transcends that minor limitation. Bringing them together and exposing Adele to a different environment occasionally, and gently, stretches her world.

Al

Eighty-three-year-old Al loved to drive or just be in the car. He prefers eating out, charming the waitresses and following the comings and goings of other "regulars" at area restaurants. His children live at a distance and get tremendous peace of mind monitoring him remotely through an innovative arrangement with strategically placed Webcams. He does not want to bother them, and, very frankly, prefers his own life in his own home rather than being segregated with "old people." He has some twinkle left in his eyes, even if his steps are slow.

Cordelia

Ninety-seven-year-old Cordelia and her 93-year-old sister, Liz, live next door to each other close to town. Cordelia joined the OSS, the CIA's precursor, during World War II and was dropped clandestinely behind enemy lines to befriend Mussolini's extended family. Lisbeth lived in Switzerland much of her adult life. Having traveled the world together since their professional lives ended and they became widows, they are enthralling dinner guests but cannot leave their homes easily without help. Their historical and literary databases are unique, and most of this potential continues to be wasted.

Lenora

Lenora, 85, now lives at a small residential-care facility in her home-town but spent her entire adult life caring for others. Then in her retirement, she cared for her husband until his death. She often cries because there is no opportunity to do for others now. She would love to volunteer looking after someone who needed her.

Fred

Fred, 85, also loved to drive, but he is at a loss as to how to pass the time since his wife was placed in a local nursing home. His kids have him over for dinner frequently but it is not enough. He visits his wife often but it is too painful for him to leave her there at the end of the visit.

Myra and Yvonne

Myra, 83, and Yvonne, 87, became friends through daily visits to their spouses in the local nursing home. They even helped out at the front desk Sunday mornings when the home was short-staffed. After their spouses' deaths, they again became isolated with no one utilizing their energy and talents.

Freda

Freda is 97 and continues to get by on her own, though she has come to dread the winter, and contemplates a move to a residential-care facility. Having been such a big part of her local community for so long, the transition will likely dull her engaging manner. She lived and worked downtown at the apothecary for most of the last century, while her husband built or renovated many of the prominent buildings in town. She still remembers every detail.

Donald and Ethel

Donald and Ethel are both 85 and are approaching their sixty-fifth wedding anniversary. They proudly insist that they are doing fine, but Ethel privately resents being confined to her bed by her arthritis, and Donald cries when she is out of sight. He is exhausted trying to keep up with the laundry from her incontinence. Some of their family is pushing for nursing home placement, which would completely devastate both of them.

Judith

Judith, 88, bounces back almost monthly to the hospital emergency room because of spells of unsteadiness and weakness that force her to reluctantly call her son for help. The family is looking to move her to a nursing home. She will go along with it so as to not bother her children, but it is far from her preference. As an avid reader still interested in the arts, and having lived and worked around the world including in Fiji, the mental constraints of her one-room existence in the nursing home with the "blah-blah ladies," as she calls them, are almost too much to bear.

Sarah

Sarah, age 67, now lives at an assisted-living facility. Despite requiring supervised care for almost a decade, she seemed too youthful and vibrant beside her older housemates. Over the last three months, however, she has taken an interest in looking after some of the other residents. Still she seeks more activity, more human connections, more engagement with art, dance, music than most of the other residents. She even hopes to fall in love again. She had majored in communication and felt that she could still contribute in a public relations role somewhere. She walks to town twice a day. She can still stack firewood or tend a garden. But she needs gentle redirection frequently during each day. Without guidance, she becomes restless, confused, and often lost.

Donna

Donna, 66, suffered a stroke involving the left hemisphere of her brain in her early sixties, and could not stay home alone. She has an expressive aphasia that impairs her ability to speak the right words most of the time. Yet, she loves to dance, paint with watercolor, and writes touching poetry. Many caregivers have trouble being around her because she is easily frustrated trying to express herself. She follows you closely at your side, afraid of getting lost or of being alone. In a small group or one-on-one, she is fine but time-consuming. Because of her needs, the assisted living home did not quite fit, and she was moved recently to a residential Alzheimer's unit. There, she initially fit, helping feed a very fragile resident, and probably recalling her former life as a nurses' aide. When that resident moved into the nursing home, Ethel was again lost. Her newfound purpose was too short-lived.

Connie

Connie, 80, lives at a picturesque farmhouse down a dirt driveway in Nobleboro. She still loves to read, act, sing, substitute teach at the high school, and shoot squirrels. She defies stereotyping. She loves to cook and entertain. She is even contemplating getting another advanced degree in psychology.

Such people represent the elder mosaic of every community. They are regular people with full former lives and remaining potential.

When you first encounter a remarkable elder, you think you have found a diamond in the rough. As you meet more and more with equally remarkable stories, you come to realize that such character and wisdom are the norm. Our elders are more like the pebbles in a stream. Each one has been individually shaped by the myriad influences of time rushing by. Each one holds a different fascination for another individual coming across that gem on a particular day in a particular light.

Our elders, like these precious stones, now need to be treasured. They now need a little assistance to live their lives to the fullest for the remainder of their days. Most wish to continue to live in their own homes. All wish to live life on their own terms. They all have adapted significantly on their own. They are not demanding. They are all capable of still contributing in significant ways to their community. If we are bold, we can see that they hold the promise for building a new network of neighbors helping neighbors, and not just more residential-care beds.

eleven

How the Maine Approach
Was Born: The Pilot Project

DEFINING A NEW SOLUTION FOR eldercare began with several brainstorming sessions involving some of my long-term-care colleagues. We focused on helping fragile elders recuperating in our skilled rehabilitation facility to return home. Gerry was one such patient whose story shaped our early thinking.

Gerry had lived a hard life. Smoking and drinking way too much, she and her husband had retired to a small home on the Pemaquid Peninsula after he retired from a Massachusetts utility company. She took care of him as long as she could, as his recurrent small strokes took more of his memory and more of his balance. Against her preferences, she relented to their daughter's insistence that he be moved to a nursing home near her in Massachusetts. Gerry's contact with her husband of fifty years was now relegated to phone calls, photos, and perhaps an annual visit. There had to be a better way, thought her nurse, Carol Richards, and me.

Gerry now clung more fiercely to her independence. She lived for her cat, a well-fed long-haired tabby. She had increasing difficulties keeping up the house, due to poor bladder control and difficulty walking as her poor leg circulation and arthritis worsened. She privately hired someone to shop once a week, to help her clean the house, and to drive her to the doctor's office every so often. She spoke more sarcastically, and it was hard to tell if this was only her lifelong sharp Irish tongue or one embittered by the struggles she was trying to endure. Because she was not officially housebound, she did not qualify for Medicare-funded home health services. She was already spending what she could afford for private help.

She fell more often, ended up in the hospital and then the rehab facility, and always insisted on returning home, as the caregiving staff cringed while admiring her pluck. She had an endearing way of connecting with the staff, with her irreverent phrases and crude humor. Although fragile, she was fully alive and not giving up. And Gerry had a unique personality and some fire in her belly that resonated with all of her caregivers.

Eventually, the nurses, neighbors, and her daughter convinced her she could not return home. They found a home for her cat. The house was sold to pay for her care for a while. Gerry was moved from the skilled unit to the long-term-care nursing unit. She never left her room. She barely left her bed. Her humor captivated a few special nurses, while the rest stayed out of reach of her clawing and spitting. She participated fully in practical jokes but not much else. She lived for several years, usually refusing her medication, and eating only when someone would take the time to sit with her. There had to be a better way.

How much extra would it really take for us to develop a system of services to help Gerry stay in her home? She did not ask for much. She did not expect much. In many ways, she did not need much. She was quite typical of so many elders: isolated, feisty, and with few options. The system had little that fit her needs in the nursing home. And it cost close to $100,000 a year to miss the mark by so much.

So I gathered together a few colleagues to brainstorm and enlarged the discussion to a forty-member senior pilot group, ages 70–95, mostly recruited from my medical practice. It became clear that the solutions needed to be infinitely flexible. Talk about herding cats. Each person had a different objective. No two could agree on the top priorities. Since the pilot group was drawn from a subset of more educated, more verbal, more successfully aging individuals, we should have expected nothing less. No one wanted to relinquish control of her life. No one wanted to give up choice. No one wanted to limit his life to just a few features.

This attitude was as frustrating as it was powerful. The pilot-group seniors were giving voice to the most essential element of an effective solution: it must address all of their diverse goals and aspirations. How do you shape an initiative that must be this individualized and this fluid? It took a few years to distill the key tenets, but most of the important features that we have incorporated into the Maine Approach were illuminated by that pilot group in 2006.

One significant realization came when Gertrude, then 95, responded to a particular version of our evolving program by saying, "Gee, Dr. Teel, that sounds wonderful. If I ever need anything, I'll let you know." I knew we had a lot more work ahead of us. "I need *you* now," I replied, "so that we can figure out how to help your neighbor." She responded affirmatively by signing up to help further that aim.

I now was zeroing in on a critical insight as to why the efforts of the health-care world to get elders to plan ahead and make changes prospectively were falling on deaf ears. These elders often have the same reaction to growing old that the rest of us do. They prefer denial: simple, stubborn, and blatant denial of what is happening in front of their eyes. But of course there is more to it.

None of us want to be continually reminded of our physical and mental limitations. It is disheartening and often disabling to be told repeatedly what you cannot do. We know that about other stages of life. Why should it be different with elders? Many analysts of successful aging point out that it is critical to maintain a positive attitude. So a survival instinct for many elders must be to reject our gloomy projections, and just go forward day-to-day, taking one's chances.

A related and equally critical corollary that surfaced was that each successfully aging person needed purpose in his or her life. Most often this purpose centered on being useful, doing something for someone else, having a reason to get up in the morning. Whether you are thirty-five or ninety-five, it feels good to do something for your neighbor. It is a central part to belonging, whatever the context:

a church, tribe, school, neighborhood, or family. Without such goals, we often lose purpose in our lives. We certainly do not live very well. With a real purpose, we become healthier, more independent, and sharper mentally, and we work harder to attain other goals.

Another important guiding principle from the pilot group days was the need to find a simple way to capture and disseminate the incredible wisdom and experience of most elders. As oral histories and photojournalist essays have shown us, there is rarely such a thing as an ordinary life. Nearly every individual who has witnessed seventy or eighty or ninety years has a wealth of interesting memories to share. But many of these memories are buried deep, and require the right combination of stimulation, curiosity, and patience to be uncovered. Moreover, most of these individuals will undervalue the importance of their accumulated experience. Unless you are a well-known celebrity who has been interviewed many times, most ordinary members of the elder community cannot imagine having any expertise that would interest another person.

Even Tom, a retired academic dean and college president for more than thirty years, would not believe that anyone would be truly interested in his lifetime of witnessing and shaping events in the tumultuous 1970s in American higher education. Given his vascular dementia, and mood disorder, it required lucky timing and proper priming to have the right lights come on. However, with a little homework, and building a little rapport, the results were well worth it. So it is with nearly everyone. How often do we read an obituary of someone we thought we knew quite well only to discover that they had lived in a place or been engaged in a job or hobby that took us by surprise? There are so many missed opportunities every day among our regular elder contacts.

It soon became clear that technology could help us not only harness this diversity but also solve various problems. If Match.com and eHarmony could create databases to find us a potential life partner, if cell phones could serve social teenagers, and if videoconferencing could connect reporters from Baghdad to the news anchor in

New York, how difficult could it be to help a woman like Gerry stay in her own home with her cat for less than the $9,000 per month she was paying to stay in the nursing unit? Over the next few years we would find out through trial and error, with unexpected discoveries along the way.

Our approach required that we build a social network among elders and facilitate ways to capture their photos, videos, and writings so they could be easily shared. If we promoted peer-to-peer contact, we stood a far better chance of getting elder interest, and simultaneously mobilizing available people resources. At first, we began assembling video "corners": three-to-five minute video clips on specific topics. Our members or volunteers would come to our office to record their thoughts, which we posted on a web-based video site called ConnectMe. They included a story corner, book corner, joke corner, and a poetry corner that were filmed using a stationary desktop computer webcam and often featured a senior narrator.

Next, our innovation utilized a small, simple video recorder called "The Flip" and uploaded segments to a website that hosted our own Elder TV. Now we are working on capturing other video content from churches, classes, speakers, and musicians, from birthday parties to holidays to regular mealtime gatherings. We are also promoting robust personal video calling, videoconferencing, and video recording with easy-to-use technology as key pieces of our regular interactions with our elders. These tools can effectively reduce loneliness and isolation in an affordable way. Moreover, they can be brought directly into anyone's home.

As our pilot developed, it became clear that a successful model must fundamentally rethink our current approach. By and large, residential-care facilities did not recognize the ongoing need for elders to have meaning in their lives. It also became clear that there is a critical ingredient to successful aging. It requires the right blend of independence and assistance, augmented by the right kind of stimulation.

Eighty-five-year-old Jenny was managing acceptably well living at home until her demanding and demented sister became ill and died. Even though Jenny regularly voiced her frustration with Edith calling her several times a day, Edith's death left Jenny alone. Shortly thereafter she moved into an assisted-living home. There she struggled with depression that we tried to medicate with antidepressants. But when pressed for what caused her frequent uncontrollable tears, she usually alluded to the fact that she had spent her whole adult life caring for others. In her retirement she cared for her husband until his death. Now without someone to care for, her life had no meaning.

At the ElderCare Network home, we could provide for all her material needs, but unless we helped her recapture some purpose, she could never be happy. She loved children too, and the home had infrequent school-children visitors. Any opportunity to give of herself to help another less fortunate is what motivated her. All the stimulation in the world could not help her find peace. Unless it was the right stimulation. And for Jenny the right stimulation needed to be doing something for others.

Soon, additional care needs required that she move from assisted living to the nursing home. Once there Jenny declined quite rapidly. That critical need to maintain independence in some fashion had also been lost. She had been successively stripped of the things that mattered most to her: connections to family, the sense of purpose that comes with doing something for someone else, and, later on, any semblance of personal control over her activities of daily living. Her decline is blamed on the progression of her underlying dementia. I am convinced, however, that a significant portion of her situation could be dramatically improved with appropriate environmental and attitudinal changes that addressed her basic underlying needs. A reality of aging is that decline does not happen in a straight line. There are good days and bad, and determining what makes a day go one way or the other is difficult, but extremely important. I've seen how difficult this is to discern, even in my own family. "Dad seemed really good the other night at the Tugboat Restaurant piano bar," noted my brother Jeff disbelievingly not too long ago. "And he was only drinking coffee, not Jameson's." Our father's ability to connect with what is going on around him varies tremendously from time to time. To date there is no discernible pattern of rest, stimulation, or location that is clearly responsible.

Rodney regained the twinkle in his eye and his easy laugh when his vivacious lifelong friends, Alice and Maddie, came to visit him at the nursing home. But the confusion was denser, the time to respond slower, than when those interactions took place in his own home. Was he succumbing to the comorbidities of his list of medical problems as the medical caregivers assume, or were there other factors at play?

Dot came to life and started playing the spoons when the right music at the right time coaxed by the right person brought her out of her shell. Mike got up, stood at attention, and saluted while singing the entire Marine Corps hymn, despite speaking very few words, and no longer remembering his wife's name. But he knew by her manner that she was special. "You are my very best friend," he would tell her.

Jean came out of her end-stage dementia nonverbal trance when her daughter played a digitally remastered recording of Jean singing an opera sixty years earlier. Janet, despite her slowly progressive profound dementia, sang all of the verses of most of the songs at the recent elder chorus called "Young At Heart" that my wife lovingly shepherds into shape.

Celia instantly goes from uncontrollable sobbing to outright delight when she sees a baby or toddler nearby. Delores knows every other resident's nighttime patterns at the assisted-living home and can help the staff sort out problems even though she regularly forgets that her parents are deceased and that her daughter recently died too.

I care for two nursing home patients who speak only a few times a month, but when they do, they are very present and engaged for most of the day. There are clearly many things going on in these aging brains that we don't understand. These individuals appear to respond to a blend of human connection, music, warmth, value, and other feel-good stuff. It is not as simple as more stimulation or less stimulation. As mentioned, it is the right stimulation, the Right Stuff. It is the proper combination of inputs that trigger a significant positive response again and again. The ability to respond, no matter how fragile the individual, never seems to be completely extinguished.

Our observation is that one's spirit is steadily worn down by the surrounding circumstances. As the therapists become increasingly apprehensive about one's safety, they convey and transfer their fears repeatedly to the patient, to the patient's family, and to the attending physician and nurse. With several of my patients whom I have seen up close, it seems that we are creating a self-fulfilling prophecy. The more we warn an individual against a behavior because they might fall, the more we reinforce their incapacity. We learned a long time ago in educational reform that for successful outcomes it is critical to have higher expectations for students. Why should it be any different with elders?

Part of what distinguishes our approach to finding the right stimulation for the elder cohort is this attitude. We are trying to identify, tease out, encourage, teach, and make commonplace these threads of liveliness that appear every day. We are trying to avoid the rote, the distant, the dispassionate, the condescending, the frustrated, the angry, and the lack of human connection that can extinguish life.

What approach is better to deal with the repetitive questions of an elder's short-term memory loss? The commonly used exasperated tone that reminds the elder that he has already asked that same question five times this morning is counterproductive, while giving him a slightly different answer each time may be a better way. For instance, "Are you going to work today?" "No, it's Saturday." A few minutes later, "Don't you have to go to work today?" "No, it's too nice a day. Let's go for a ride." Or "No, I'd rather spend it with you." Or "No, I don't. Will you help me with this puzzle or this project?" Or "No, I don't. Can you tell me about the time you went to . . .?"

While this exercise may seem silly, it's a necessary technique for helping engage and stimulate an elder with short-term memory loss.

As we zero in on many of the tough situations highlighted by our Maine work, it inevitably raises questions as to how the Maine Approach will deal with the toughest elder customers. As we push the envelope further, I am more convinced that very few need to be excluded. Many have doubted that we can serve a large number of frail elders with this method, especially those with complex needs. Our experience to date proves otherwise. Many residential-care developers want to focus on the easier customers. After our experience of the last five years, I am not sure where the boundary is that separates appropriate candidates for our approach.

I believe we were able to see these themes more clearly because of the intense personal lens we were shining on our elders. We were looking for the nonmedical, the human interaction, and we are finding it.

twelve

The Maine Approach Menu

MY PILOT PROJECT LED ME TO VARIOUS local experiments over five years. We crafted different services that we operated under the names "LincMe," at the beginning, and then later as "Elder Power," and we have further refined the services offered to other communities under Full Circle America affiliates. Building upon our experience with those programs, we developed the full menu of services that we thought critical to eldercare, and we called it the Maine Approach. Eventually, we settled upon three different service bundles, which we called Basic, Premium, and Deluxe packages. All our participants—we call them "members"—can choose a package that includes varying levels of support from this menu:

- a personal advocate/consultant
- telephone and video phone calls, usually from an elder volunteer
- Guardian 911 emergency-response system
- remote video monitoring
- volunteer home visits
- transportation or errand services (frequency varies by level chosen)
- personal weekly planner
- monthly community activity calendar
- video calling
- semiannual mental health assessments
- access to our website and e-mail services

- all members are able to volunteer to help others
- membership in the "Home Away From Home" program to reduce loneliness and generate supplemental income

The higher monthly packages incorporate targeted at-home personal support designed to give regular on-site human touch in addition to the robust technology-based support.

Additional personal support services can be added to any package at $25 per hour to meet more frequent needs for transportation, errands, shopping, meal preparation, laundry, bathing, and home repairs. Our first effort is to try and provide these services through an unpaid volunteer. Only when a volunteer is not available, or the task requires special skills, do we send a paid employee or provider. Our objective is to try to keep the costs low, not pump them up.

Right from the beginning, we have emphasized choice. Members eligible for a feature opt in rather than being forced to accept every offering. This is very important since we are building a relationship. I expect that many potential members may have unappealing preconceived notions about elder services. Many may have had difficulty just getting up the nerve to call or visit or seek information or help. These decisions are for them monumental; they are personal and demand that a significant amount of trust be placed with an organization.

In the old paradigm, most elders would not explore a residential housing option until a crisis developed and doctor or family insisted upon a change. Such a response was understandable given the combination of denial and lack of choice. No matter what our age, many of us prefer to ignore obvious impending events because we have no good choices, or we must face up to a reality we find odious. The Maine Approach is different. It reengages you in living, champions what you can still do with what you have left in the tank, and gives you some very new tools, like video calling, videoconferencing, and video recording, to help you maintain independence, to empower you to make your own social circle, and to make a difference in your community.

In table 12.1, the main features of the three packages are displayed so that a prospective member or his or her family may compare and contrast them.

For those that sign up for a year of service, there are no initial sign-up fees, evaluation fees, or other up-front charges, and all of the

PACKAGE FEATURES	BASIC	PREMIUM	DELUXE
PERSONAL MEMBER ADVOCATE	✔	✔	✔
VIDEO/TELEPHONE CALLS (daily)	✔	✔	✔
ERRAND SERVICE		2×/month	weekly
VIDEOPHONE: ASUS/VOSKY/LOGITECH	✔	✔	✔
FCA WEBSITE (full access)	✔	✔	✔
MEMBER CARE CENTER (M–F 9–5)			
WEEKLY PLANNER (unlimited updates)	✔	✔	✔
MONTHLY ACTIVITY CALENDAR (with reminders; activities may have extra charges)	✔	✔	✔
DEEP-SUPPORT SERVICES (transportation, repairs, errands, shopping, meals, laundry, bath		$25/hr	$25/hr
VOLUNTEERING (in community or at home)	✔	✔	✔
WEBCAMS/Gateway (for video monitoring)	1 pan/tilt camera	pan/tilt + stationary	pan/tilt + stationary
SENSORS (for door, motion detection, temperature, or water-leak detection)	temperature sensor	temperature sensor	motion detector/ door/temp. sensor
VIDEO MONITORING (hourly/continuous)		from $150/month	from $150/month
HOME HEALTH (at-home weight, pulse, blood pressure, oxygen saturation)		✔	✔
MENTAL HEALTH ASSESSMENT (family wellness toolkit to help with depression, anxiety, cognition, attention, behavior, or functional problems)	every 6 months	every 6 months	every 6 months
MONTHLY SUMMARY (to family/ doctor)		✔	✔
"HOME AWAY FROM HOME" NETWORK		✔	✔

Table 12.1. The Maine Approach menu of services resulted from local experiments, pilot projects, and close attention to the true needs of elders. Pricing shown here is from April 2011.

equipment required to supply the services at each level is included in the monthly charge. We prefer to bill through a credit card for simplicity and to maintain our cash flow. However, where requested we will submit paper invoices and wait for checks.

What follows is more detail regarding several of the services described in the menu grid that have not been previously discussed.

The Personal Member Advocate

This person is the member's main advocate and can be a friend, family member, the person who made the referral, a volunteer, another more experienced member, a phone-tree captain, or a staff person. We sometimes refer to the personal advocate as a member's guardian angel. The advocate's duties include contacting the member as often as appropriate and building a flexible, natural relationship based around the member's needs. When the advocate discovers that a member may need or want a change in services, that information is conveyed to the affiliate manager for follow-up.

Marie is an example of a personal member advocate. She is a retiree volunteer who works in our office. She speaks with member Gertrude regularly and occasionally transports her to an appointment or runs an errand for her. Marie then uses her knowledge and insight about Gertrude to recommend other services for her as well as making sure that when we do our monthly service review, we do so accurately.

Telephone Checks

Depending upon the level of support requested, we have volunteers make telephone calls to each member. We recommend calls at least once a day, but often a follow-up call is needed. We have found our members prefer to ease into this. The relationship develops slowly, with either the new member calling us, or more commonly, one of our telephone captains initially calling a new member a few times a week. The content is meant to be fluid and friendly, and private unless the member seeks otherwise, or the phone captain detects some actionable information.

Sally is a great phone captain. As a retired social worker who keeps up avidly with what is going on in the world of news, weather, and sports, she has a fabulous phone manner that endears her to each member she calls. When she recently visited friends out of state over Christmas, she brought her phone list with her so as not to shirk her responsibility. Having lost most of her sight, she regularly expresses her gratitude to be made to feel useful again. She sure is. This is an example of elder-to-elder volunteerism that helps to manage costs while helping the caller and the person called.

Judy is another exceptional telephone captain. Having been a personal caregiver throughout our community until her own health failed, she truly looks forward to making her daily calls. Even when she was admitted to the hospital recently, she brought her phone list with her, and made her calls from her hospital bed. This is the kind of dedication that makes the Maine Approach tick.

Videophones

With the advent of stand-alone, touch-screen, Wi-Fi-enabled videophones, our approach to daily contact with elder members is changing. Providing all members with a videophone and creating an elder videophone social network is our current target. The videophone is a gateway device not only to connect better to family and friends, but also to give back by becoming a video buddy to someone that that elder can serve. Distance is no longer an obstacle. Whether a young student needs additional positive reinforcement, or a single mom needs another virtual grandparent, or an isolated elder needs peer support, such help is now a push button away. And our elder members can once again have added purpose to their lives.

Video Spot Checking

We utilize web-enabled pan-and-tilt cameras that are ID and password protected, but accessible to authorized family and staff from wherever Internet service is available. Our members and their families have tremendous peace of mind that an elder is safe and secure, and that someone local and dedicated to their well-being is assisting them.

Depending upon the level of support selected by the member, video spot checks are performed on a schedule and as needed when there is concern about the member. The checks are performed by one of our paid or volunteer staff. With our current technology each check is logged and any "actionable information" is conveyed to the office manager or health-care professional on call. The phrases "every picture tells a story" or "a picture is worth a thousand words" absolutely convey the value of these cameras to the members of the network.

Roger is our video volunteer extraordinaire. Disabled by a motorcycle accident many years ago, his employment options have been severely limited. Yet his active, healthy mind and caring disposition have made him an ideal person for this task. He represents what most vocational-rehabilitation counselors desire for their clients, a computer-based job that can be performed from home. But to Roger, it is considerably more than that. He has been given an opportunity to be of tremendous value to a vulnerable and often invisible population of fragile at-home elders. The meaning that this role has given to his own life is incalculable.

Like all our volunteers, he takes his job very seriously. Even though he has not met most of the members he diligently checks, he knows them better than most family members. The motion-driven video snapshots tell him at a glance whether anything is out of place in the home scene surveyed. Similarly, a member following his or her usual routine contributes to a daily assessment that all is well.

Since we monitor primarily the kitchen, with all the shots time-stamped, such things as dishes in the sink or not, newspaper or mail on the kitchen table or not, visitors at the kitchen table, or the member getting something out of the refrigerator, all tell a great deal about the day.

These snapshots provide a body of work that surpasses anything most residential-care facilities can offer. They rival and sometimes exceed the information provided by in-home caregivers since the information is unfiltered, and candid, not shaped by the interaction between member and caregiver. For many members, this surveillance is much less intrusive than agency caregivers being in their homes many hours a day.

Most members do not find these video spot checks an invasion of privacy. As a matter of fact, many members find great comfort in knowing someone is looking out for them. Most cameras come with privacy buttons. All cameras can be easily draped with a napkin to afford immediate privacy. Moreover, the images are not being broadcast indiscriminately, but are only available to authorized individuals with the password. Most images are erased on a daily basis; the only ones that are archived or saved are representative shots that we keep on file to guide us to detect changes in members over time or to confirm that a scheduled paid visit or service was performed.

Compare this inconvenience to the far larger loss of privacy that results from moving into a double bedroom in a residential-care facility, sharing a bathroom, bureau, and closet with a complete stranger, and being tended to by a constantly changing staff of caregivers. To challenge the contention that Big Brother is watching, I offer the following. Despite the Orwellian connotation, many big brothers historically have been a welcome protector. It is also important to remember that every level of support, and monitoring, is by the choice and consent of the member. And their decisions can be reversed at their discretion.

So far, video care of members has detected falls, and led to prompt staff responses, averting many trips to the hospital. Other times, power outages and furnace failures have been detected and addressed. This tool also provides to us a well-documented means of quality assurance. We can see for ourselves whether our staff member or volunteer has arrived when expected and how long they have remained. Substandard performers are easily weeded out. Once we identified a private caregiver (not one of ours thank goodness) stealing from a member, which led to the return of the stolen money.

Most importantly, the warmth and richness of the images imme-diately draw one into the lives of the members, and extend that same feeling to distant family members. They also give extraordi-nary detail that can often identify changes before a major problem develops. So, despite the initial reluctance of many older individuals to embrace such a new idea, it only takes one incident for a camera to prove its value. As the Maine Approach emphasizes choice, no member is required to have such a service. We are confident that with time, as a member's trust of us and our approach grows, he or she will see the wisdom of this feature.

Home Visits

Home visits are an essential feature of the Maine Approach. No sophisticated technology can take the place of such personal interac-tion, what we call "touches." The home visit may be from a nurse, another staff person, the personal advocate, or a volunteer. Often the visitors are also members fulfilling their own desire to be helpful. All are selected because of their people skills and dedication to the mission. Because of the uniqueness of our approach, we are able to attract the best from every community.

Carol Richards and Janet Yates, our two exceptional nurses, do many of our home visits and exemplify another important theme. Generally speaking, and just like the rest of us, nurses too are very disgruntled with the current health-care system. I deal with them every day in all sorts of situations and settings. Most nurses do not think the current model serves older individuals properly. They sincerely wish that the goals of service, genuine helping, and personal connections that attracted them to nursing were more deeply valued by the health-care institutions for which they work. They have seen regulatory and financial concerns erode all other values. They are easily attracted to our approach as it truly represents why they and their colleagues went into the profession.

The frequency of visits is partially determined by the package chosen. The length of the visit is not predetermined but generally lasts from fifteen minutes to an hour depending upon the situation. The content of the visit is similarly unscripted. But the goal is primarily to see that each member is getting what she expects and needs, and to work together with the member to solve problems arising from any unmet need or desire. Often the need is as small as taking out the trash or getting the mail.

Home visits can be used to teach a member a new skill. They can be used to initiate a video call to a family member or friend. They are used to share video highlights from a recent event on the Elder TV site or further explain the social networking features.

Together with the errand and transportation services, the visits provide opportunities to grow the relationship, and to reduce the loneliness and isolation of members. Sometimes including another member in a home visit provides mutual benefit. Several members of our community have known each other from their earlier days, but owing to declining health or other reasons, have lost touch. They now welcome the opportunity to be reconnected by our staff person or a volunteer. Carol and Janet have helped orchestrate and execute several small dinner parties and small group outings.

Transportation and Errand Service

Elders often cite transportation as their most challenging obstacle to home living. Whether it is getting to doctor appointments, grocery shopping, or running necessary errands, the tasks associated with getting out of the house become formidable when declining vision, balance, and strength interfere. Difficulties dealing with such basic needs preclude rekindling any interest in other community events such as movies, theater, music, sports, church, and service organizations. Combating rampant loneliness and isolation among elders in our community mandates addressing transportation. It is an essential piece of any effort to help elders stay in their own homes and to renew their involvement with family, friends, and community.

We have included a basic level of transportation service within our packages, and more extensive services are available to meet the needs of members who are required to make multiple trips or appointments each week. Ideally family, church groups, and friends will meet the transportation needs related to health care, so our focus can be on getting the member out of the house for some fun. We feel philosophically that a disproportionate amount of transportation resources in most communities is devoted to medical issues.

Volunteer Opportunities

As I have noted throughout this book, central to the Maine Approach is seeing our elders as a hidden resource for both affordable labor and volunteer effort. Once recognized as capable of making a difference in so many ways in their community, it is only natural to design a program around the abilities of our elders. The arithmetic is compelling. If just 10–15 percent of the over-65 population will contribute four hours a week to a meaningful activity, the resultant labor force would meet all of the needs of every elder.

We are not talking about token busy work here. We have identified the individual triggers that cause elders and their families to seek residential-care options for their loved ones. Then we defined the ways in which many other elders and community members can address these triggers. We continue to implement our findings. But it is abundantly clear that if we identify the specific tasks that need doing, we can then delegate these to the appropriate members of the elder community, thereby fundamentally changing the outcome of residential-care placement in many cases.

Most seniors desire to continue to make meaningful contributions to the communities around them. When I spoke to the Pemaquid Cooperative Ministry's community outreach forum in March, 2010, more than a dozen ninety-plus-year-olds in attendance signed up to volunteer to help their neighbors in the approach we outlined. It was truly remarkable to see so many elders who are not commonly sought out, commit to participate. Clearly our approach resonated loudly with their sense of what needs to be done.

Overall, as I watched our Maine Approach team struggle to reinvent a workable and affordable home-care support system, I began to realize that what drove us forward was an appreciation of our patients that went well beyond their physical challenges. Our volunteers and core trained staff too had this special gift that allowed them to appreciate the whole person and his or her enduring value.

I say this is a gift because it shows a remarkable quality in our staff and volunteers to truly appreciate each human being before them while in the process becoming more connected to their community. I realized that the volunteers we could most count on were the ones that had this ability. And that tied into a more practical realization that in order to recruit and retain the hundreds of thousands of volunteers of all ages that would be required to serve tens of millions of elders in the immediate future, we would have to help all those involved tap into that inner quality of goodwill and commitment toward our older neighbors, seen above and in many other examples.

Emergency Call Buttons

Of all the emergency call services commercially available, a Lifeline Button probably is the most well known. Even so, it has often taken a lot of convincing to get elder loved ones to agree to get one. Once they have one, many do not use it because they leave it on the bureau or in the bathroom. Others do not want to bother anyone, or they do not think their particular problem is serious enough to end up going to the hospital. Or they fear it might be serious and try to ignore the problem. So they do not push the button. Still others push it quite frequently not for help but for conversation. Even a stranger at a call center is a welcome social interaction for many deprived of human connections. A Lifeline Button costs $40–$50 per month.

With these factors in mind, we instead use and are happy with LogicMark products called Guardian 911 and Freedom Alert. The advantages are that these buttons have no recurring monthly fees. They can be purchased outright with a one-time cost and then are owned by the customer. We have chosen to include them in every package we offer.

Guardian 911 and Freedom Alert systems have several other advantages. The speaker is on the device you carry rather than back at the base station. This allows the wearer to talk directly to the call center representative rather than trying to talk from a separate room or even through a closed door. Their latest product, the Freedom Alert button, has three modes on the back of the base station: direct 911 notification, sequential dialing of four programmable numbers, or the programmable sequence followed by an automatic 911 call. This button fits many circumstances where a frail elder cannot get to or use a telephone easily. It can become their version of a cordless receiver, albeit limited to one specific number or sequence. So we have incorporated their features into our packages, knowing that they play a role. With the passive monitoring available with our webcams and motion sensors, they make our packages the most comprehensive available.

Weekly Planner

This simple tool came out of our experience where home health agencies routinely scheduled their visits according to their availability and not that of the customer. It not only was insensitive to the client's life but also many elders would not do anything else that day other than wait for their visitor. The form we use allows us to have a pretty good read at a glance of the individual elder's life and routine. We can help them plan an outing or tailor a volunteer visit to fill in a slow part of their week. We can remind them of upcoming events or appointments. We can share this information with the phone-tree captain, our nurse, and the video spot checker to coordinate their roles.

Monthly Activity Calendar

A monthly activity calendar is compiled at least a week in advance of the start of every month. It merges the community calendar provided by the local newspaper with that provided by the senior center, the residential-care homes, and public radio. It attempts to highlight those activities that may interest our members.

This calendar is more than a bulletin. We seek to have every member attend at least one and preferably two nonmedical events outside of their homes each month. We have found that the positive impact of attendance at such events can last weeks. We call this afterglow effect a "bounce," and it can make all the difference.

Our personal advocates, phone captain, home visitors, and other volunteers are all charged with helping identify events that each member would like to participate in. Next, it is their follow-up task to help implement that member's attendance at their selected events. We will help with tickets and transportation. We offer reminders. It is in keeping with our mission to engage elders in events going on in their community.

FULL CIRCLE ACTIVITY TABLE
• GO OUT TO LUNCH: Monday at the elementary school / Tuesday at the high school / Wednesday at senior center / Thursday at area churches / Friday at area restaurants
• HOST/JOIN A SUPPER CLUB: Socialize monthly for the fun of it. You are the host once a year. Help with preparation and clean-up provided.
• TAKE A CLASS /ATTEND A LECTURE: Senior college / adult ed / area speakers
• TAKE IN A MOVIE LOCALLY: Monday at Skidompha Library in the evening / Thursday afternoon at someone's home.
• HELP SOMEONE WITH EASY REPAIRS: From repairing a lamp or a picture frame to a storm window project.
• BABYSIT FOR A FEW HOURS A WEEK: Help give a young mother a break.
• HOST A YOUNG STUDENT FOR A FEW HOURS A WEEK: Provide a quiet place to do homework.
• BE A COMPANION TO AN OLDER NEIGHBOR FOR A FEW HOURS A WEEK
• HIRE A YOUTH TO DO SOME YARD WORK FOR YOU
• TEACH A YOUTH TO BAKE COOKIES OR SEW ON A BUTTON
• JOIN A VOLUNTEER EVENT CREW: Help local nonprofits host their occasional events.
• OFFER A RIDE TO SOMEONE ELSE / OR PICK UP AN ORDER WHEN YOU SHOP OR RUN ERRANDS
• JOIN A CATERING SERVICE: Dig out a favorite recipe to make a home-cooked meal for someone else.
• JOIN THE COMMUNITY CALL CENTER: Make a few phone calls to remind someone to take her medicine, or encourage her to join a local activity, or just chat.

Table 12.2. Our staff uses this lineup of suggested activities to help members plan at least two nonmedical events outside their home each month.

Mental Health Assessment

This Maine Approach feature grew out of our desire to demonstrate the value and power of what we were doing. Empirically, it made sense that if we could improve the rest of an older individual's life he or she would be happier, need less medical care, and be healthier longer. But we needed to find a way to track such data in a way that was not too cumbersome.

The ASEBA scoring system pioneered by Dr. Achenbach and the Vermont Center for Children, Youth, and Family provided the tool we were looking for. It has an Older Adult Behavioral Checklist that can be scored by our members or their families. It scores each member in the domains of depression, anxiety, cognition, attention, behavior, and physical functioning. We have chosen to offer it twice a year.

Monthly Summary

In keeping with our desire to regularly prove ourselves to our customers, we send a brief summary, on request, to the individual, a family member, or the individual's primary care physician. It is a simple summary of the monthly highlights of that member and the service package they have received.

Respite Opportunities

Respite care is a concept whereby individuals, while desiring to stay in their own homes or with extended-family members in their homes, often need temporary room and board when their primary caregiving family member is unavailable due to work, illness, hobbies, children, or vacation. As a concept, respite care is gaining traction, but capacity is lacking in most communities. We have successfully tested a "Home Away From Home" Program whereby older homeowners may contribute spare rooms to our network pool for respite care, day care, and additional social networking.

Very few elders desire to be in a larger residential-care facility, and very few require such a concentration of services. Most desire to stay in their own homes, and prefer respite care in a homelike setting when needed. Many elders have downsized in their own homes, closing off or not using large parts of the home. Matching needs is very possible if there is a trusted facilitator and problem solver for such a network.

Our evolving Home Away From Home concept provides an affordable solution. Elder homeowners can do as much or as little hosting as they desire. We link together this network of spare bedrooms utilizing digital technologies and support services to convert the underutilized capacity into a new revenue stream for elder homeowners and an additional care option for the community. Within two weeks of proposing such a network at a community meeting, we had thirty rooms offered with very few questions asked.

Although this service is still in the trial phase, we believe the Home Away From Home network can also be an inexpensive, multipurpose alternative for those whose needs are not easily served in our current health-care system. Such cases might involve:

- those not quite ready to return home from the hospital unsupervised but no longer requiring expensive inpatient care;
- fragile individuals seen in the emergency room but not deemed to be a third-party-payer "covered" admission;
- individuals needing a few days of additional strengthening prior to returning home from either hospital or the SNF units, having met targets but still not quite safe;
- individuals requiring "preps" for upcoming surgeries that are difficult for those living alone; they used to be admitted overnight before a procedure;
- individuals who need testing to further evaluate a problem for which an admission is no longer allowed;

- frail spouses of those admitted to hospital while
  their loved one recovers;
- those awaiting "placement" in long-term care;
- elder abuse situations where the removal from the
  home is required for the safety of the patient and a
  safe place to stay is needed.

At first glance, it may appear that many of these situations are beyond the capability of at-home elders to handle. I urge you to think again. It requires good screening, back-up technology, and personal support services from the community. The payoff for all concerned is immeasurable. More to the point, there are no other ready and affordable alternatives.

While there are other private-pay services, and even many charitable organizations who can meet some of these needs, we aspire to offer them all in a well-organized fashion and at an affordable cost. There has been considerable trial and error, and there will be more to come. But we now have a working model.

This in-depth look at the menu of our Maine Approach shows how the insights outlined earlier have been translated into a rich but reproducible system to enable most elders to stay in their own homes. It also empowers them, and gives them the tools to remain active in their communities, connected to family and friends, and to maintain meaning and value in their lives.

• thirteen •

Connecting Elders to Each Other and to Caregivers through Technology

The Maine Approach began with the not so modest ambition to fundamentally change the way our society values and cares for its most experienced members. We desperately needed options for elders to remain fully engaged with family, friends, community, and interests—promoting blended independence and interdependence. Our goal was to bring the richness of each community into each individual's life and to allow elders to share the richness of their lives with others as they saw fit. Our approach changes the landscape from the current context where elder interaction focuses primarily on pills, fall prevention, urinary incontinence, and constantly reminding them of all of their limitations. It is that context that leaves a large cohort of elders to simply pass the time waiting to die.

We have long been a youth-oriented culture with retirement often heralding a transition time into a sort of limbo after a brief flurry of vigorous volunteering. However, with our steadily increasing longevity has also come a dramatic improvement in general geriatric health, ushering in decades of living for many with reasonably well-controlled chronic conditions.

So if we live for twenty or thirty years after retirement, what are our roles in society? Only recently, a few pockets of vigorous seniors have taken matters into their own hands in such diverse places as Beacon Hill Village in Boston, Staying Put in New Canaan, Connecticut, and senior-driven initiatives in Palo Alto, California, and Alexandria, Virginia. Most seniors want to stay in their own homes. Most would prefer to remain involved in cultural and community activities. Surprisingly, most grossly undervalue their own accumulated wisdom and experience. They would repeatedly downplay the importance of any contributions they could still make to our society. Those around them, however, regularly marvel at the richness of their lives and are enchanted by the encounters. All of us yearn for more intergenerational contacts, and few of us have much opportunity for them.

Most importantly, most elders find the options for long-term care both unpalatable and unaffordable, and all agree that combating loneliness and isolation is the most critical component of successful aging. Achieving such a goal requires addressing the impact of widely dispersed family and friends, and reducing the impact of declining vision, hearing, ambulation, and dexterity. It requires championing widespread interaction between the rich untapped resource of experience and wisdom that elders possess with the other broad segments of our society that yearn for such connections. It requires harnessing the potential of technology and utilizing ingenuity to knit together the various elements of such an endeavor.

Essentially, it requires providing the tools for lifelong networking. In Maine, we decided to assess what technological options could help elders stay connected to family and friends, be monitored if they so chose, and network with each other to create an elder-assisted care community—not just an assisted-care community for elders. Like the ubiquitous Verizon ads, when you sign up, you get a lot of people behind the scene that are available to you, but you choose how and what pieces to employ. As the AT&T slogan "Your World Delivered" implies: you must participate in an important way, at least by voicing your opinion as to what is important to you.

Again through pilot programs with a few dozen elders, LincMe has distilled the necessary technological components of a successful model and has put them to use in the Maine Approach. One of the first things we found, of course, was that the "people" part of the model needed to be emphasized more than the technology.

Technology scared most elders and, until only recently, it often intimidated their adult children, too.

We realized early on that a fully functional people-and-technology program would need to allow each member to choose the features that are most desirable or most necessary now, and to modify the choices as often as necessary as individual circumstances change. A lifelong network has unlimited potential connections. It incorporates human and technological elements. It is fluid and is also simultaneously local and international. It has no age boundaries, though people with different needs and abilities may require different adaptation, but overall, it is intergenerational at its core. It must also incorporate elements of safety and security. It must acknowledge and address the changes in our bodies and minds as we age. Yet the approach must remove the hurdles that inhibit continued and full participation in our society.

Another intrinsic aspect of the lifelong network is that it is I-centered yet not selfish, while the individual defines the intricacy of the weave. Each individual takes certain responsibility for accessing and searching for the appropriate features for his or her needs. The word "network" suggests various synonyms like "tracks," "circuitry," "channels," "system," "labyrinth," "arrangement," "weave," "mesh." There are many connotations and forms to this lifelong network. As "I" begin to explore and employ the options available to "me," I become more empowered, more confident, more in control of my own life. As I am encouraged, I can walk further. I eat healthier. I do more for myself. As I am empowered to take back my life, I am less lonely. I laugh more. I contribute more each day. I am no longer alone and invisible.

The value that this paradigm shift brings to our whole society is almost incalculable. If we can reallocate large amounts of resources, both human and capital, the benefits are widespread. If we can harness the vast potential of this large demographic segment of our population and convert them from either recipients or bystanders to full participants, the possibilities are endless. Further, in most communities, if our approach engages only 10 percent of those over sixty-five years old to contribute only four hours a week to a meaningful endeavor, it makes this entity the people equivalent of the largest employer in the area. Do the math. Try it in your community. You will be astounded.

So this vision eventually emerged. It did not come out fully developed. It took time and experience to rework it over and over again. In the meantime, I had enough collaborators to help shape that vision, enough pioneering customers to try it out, and enough volunteers and staff to help implement it. But in the end, we came up with a core group of services that meet various needs.

First, we gathered existing technology and community resources and bundled them in convenient arrays. Video-calling and video-messaging software applications like ConnectMe, MSN Video Messenger, SightSpeed, and Skype opened up the power of video communication to everyone having an Internet connection, webcam, and monitor or television. Elders could send and receive video from new grandchildren, about pets' antics, or just stay in touch with friends.

Through videoconferencing, elders can participate in coffee klatches, book groups, and sewing/quilting/knitting groups, from their own homes. Minds and bodies remained active through story corners, poetry corners, book corners, and joke corners, as well as art, dance, exercise, and cooking sessions. Formerly active members can still participate in meetings of the Lions Club, Rotary, Chamber of Commerce, and Knights of Columbus even if they no longer drive at night. One can video-stream local speakers, musical performances, science fairs, and church services into any home if transportation, ambulation, or time constraints interfere. Video content can also be gathered via mini-camcorders, uploaded to the website, and appropriately indexed.

Our small group of sixty current members who have used these programs point to their ease of use and broad application. We have collected some priceless video clips, and have used the various applications for novice users in nursing homes, assisted-living residences, and independent-living apartments. We have also done our share of technology advising, purchase and reselling, and local-service delivery along the way.

These same tools allow us to care for each other remotely too. We cannot ignore the enormous peace of mind that safety and health-care access and control provide for all individuals and their families. Products like infrared motion sensors and surveillance cameras from AT&T and Xanboo allow us to monitor members in their homes. These tools let us supplement the attention of family members, neighbors, and traditional service providers, and open the door for many new service relationships including peer-to-peer care. We are also seeing a wave of new products that can serve to expand the current monitoring capabilities and reduce the cost of such technology.

We began by placing a variety of these items in the homes of a small group of local elders. Over time we have blended this technology with focused on-site care determined by the individualized needs of each member, often identified and refined by the technology itself. Where necessary the video monitoring can be essentially 24/7. But in the interest of cost, efficiency, and privacy, it rarely needs to be. We are always fine-tuning the interpretive component and networking with other compatible partners. The peace of mind generated for family members is enormous. The richness of the detail and the diversity of components and options available are in stark contrast to what current residential care offers.

Of course, the relevant technology is rapidly changing and regularly offering new opportunities to incorporate more features. Our current approach has been to incorporate components from existing companies with readily available product and support and also a track record of innovation and sustainability. The components must be affordable, reliable, and broadly available. They must be easy to use by the target population. Our focus is to integrate them into a service umbrella that tries to meet the vast and varied wants and needs outlined in chapter 12. Within the next year, we'll need to build our own fully-integrated software system to seamlessly provide the turnkey operation we envision offering each local affiliate.

People will always be the primary ingredient. The people of the network need to be committed to each other and the goals clearly outlined. This is a service business to an often vulnerable population. The integrity, sense of personal accountability, and dedication of all serving in the organization must be the highest priority at all times. Too often the focus is on the gadget rather than the people and the process. Our elder advocates and support staff must embody the cardinal principle of genuinely enjoying and respecting our elders, and be committed to empowering them to continue as independent, active members of their community.

As all of the monitoring devices are Internet driven, sufficient bandwidth is essential. Fortunately, DSL, fiber optics, satellites, cellular technology, Wi-Fi, and other repeaters/relays make Internet availability much broader than even a year ago, and likely to be almost universally available and affordable soon. Time Warner Cable has been very accommodating to us in Maine over the last thirty-six months by arranging installation on short notice, waving long-term contracts, providing modems at no charge, and generally being very service oriented.

On the hardware side we have experimented with a variety of products, and the options are expanding rapidly. Netbooks have arrived to provide enough computing power and connectivity to meet most of our needs in a very portable and affordable unit. Touch screens are now more broadly available and often very affordable. Many manufacturers are making Skype video applications a built-in feature on their televisions. Netbooks with a VGA plug to connect adequate, cheap computing power easily to a large-screen television and computer-connected TVs are rapidly merging the two media. Many manufacturers are bringing Skype and other video applications to many cell phone models. Cost, customer acceptance, convenience, and corporate positioning are all in rapid-change mode.

Plug-and-play stand-alone video phones are quickly emerging

as an essential component of our brand-new, ready-to-grow elder social network. Using a seven-inch touch screen featuring Skype video applications, products from ASUS and Vosky have built-in Wi-Fi connections and "always-on" features to provide friendly user interfaces for technology-naïve elders. Some are now even incorporating digital picture frames with e-mail delivery capabilities. The opportunity to bring elders easily into two-way video contact with other elders and other family members with the touch of a finger is phenomenal. The ability to simply modify loneliness and isolation while circumventing the troublesome mobility and transportation obstacles is huge.

At present, personal home computers and "smart" cell phones with video capability provide options for almost every budget and offer view-ability and portability choices.

One can add an ever larger flat-panel monitor with a built-in webcam and microphone and in the process dramatically upgrade what many older people possess while providing the other components for the software and programs. Group purchasing and private-label branding will improve upon the price further. Integrating the member's existing television is desirable to encourage easy adoption.

Google TV and the Logitech set-top box have just made a smooth merger between basic cable TV services and the incredible power and diversity of the Internet and web-based programming applications. These first-generation devices already allow the older individual, from the comfort of the easy chair in their own living room, to quickly and easily switch from watching a TV program to answering a big-screen video call from a family member, a friend, or a caregiver to interacting with one's own local social network features via an Internet home-page portal. As we are able to write customized applications for the diverse needs of at-home elders, the utility of this multifunctionality will amplify rapidly.

Now for the software. Skype continues to show up in more and more places. Once a family has been introduced to the amazing added value of video calling, it is hard to think of going back to plain long-distance phone calls with close family and friends. It is a free basic download that allows everyone to try it without obligation. A nine-user multiparty video conferencing feature is available for a low monthly fee.

I am also very excited about the richness of advances in video calling, video messaging, and videoconferencing generally. They have plans that offer unlimited video calling anywhere in the world with the ability to record the live call when desired, unlimited five-minute-length video messaging with storage indefinitely on their servers, multiparty videoconferencing that is an easy three-click process rather than a complicated hosting process. I believe it would serve many of our intended senior social interactions; it also adds an easy interface with landline telephones and has compatibility with Microsoft and Apple users so that we can include the Maine school children and many college and professional users with whom we have had difficulty working in the recent past.

A big key to our success has been our remote video-monitoring package from Xanboo and AT&T. It offers reliable webcams, motion sensors, temperature sensors, and other smart-home devices connected to a controller that keeps information files on their server and has a secure, reliable, and user-friendly interface for our staff and member families to access. We have employed their products since 2006, and we are impressed with the quality of images, the flexibility of the software and storage options (complete with the ability to make narrative notations), and the speed and connectivity from anywhere in the world. We are continuing to discover applications for their products. The information can be accessed and options managed from any computer or compatible cell phone anywhere. Starting with products originally designed for remote monitoring of vacation homes or nanny cams, we have made them granny cams. Their ability to design a combined home security and personal health-monitoring system makes this program very attractive.

From a basic starter kit (with one camera and one door sensor) to a deluxe starter kit (with two cameras, including one pan/tilt and one door sensor), and adding extra door/window sensors, wireless motion sensors, a wireless event-alarm signal, with optional wireless power controls to turn lights and appliances on and off remotely, we can offer a very slick personal monitoring and home security system. These options cost much less than the basic systems from ADT, GE, and Brinks, and are far more informative and comprehensive.

They also allow video checking from anywhere in the world via cell or computer, the ability to arm and disarm the various components remotely as well, and the tremendous flexibility to capture and store still photos all day, every day, at desired intervals. If one desired 24/7 continuous video recording from any or all cameras, a DVR with a 30–60-day capacity can be added.

Another unique software provider for us has been QuietCare. It offers a series of wireless activity sensors that learn a person's daily living patterns, tabulate each day's events, detect variations in patterns, automatically send out emergency alerts as well as daily e-mail summaries to designated caregivers and/or family members, and is professionally monitored 24/7. The password-protected activity reports on their website are continuously updated and can be accessed by family or caregivers at anytime anywhere. The information is collected wirelessly by the controller in the person's home and transmitted through a shared phone line. No Internet access is required in the person's home for this type of monitoring.

Wireless sensors are generally placed in each room as well as the refrigerator and medicine cabinet. Let's say you are monitoring your father as I have been monitoring mine. The data collected assesses whether dad got up and out of the bedroom this morning; whether there is a strong possibility that he has fallen in the bathroom; whether he is preparing meals regularly or remembering to take medications on time or at all; whether he is sleeping well; whether he is getting less active during the day; whether his home is too hot or cold; how many times he gets up at night to use the bathroom. All of these events are recorded to the minute, summarized in graphic form, or capable of being analyzed singly or compared to the week or month's pattern. By pattern recognition and patient knowledge, a lot of additional information can be inferred that a daily conversation alone might not provide.

Information like this doesn't replace human contact, but it can improve the decisions made with an elder, or—in worst cases—on his or her behalf. The detail is far more exact and comprehensive than the best skilled nursing facility can provide. The algorithms summarize the daily activity according to red lights that indicate a possible emergency and generate an immediate call, yellow lights that indicate changes in behavior that may require further investigation, and green lights that signal safe situations.

To my surprise, the information I've collected on my dad so unobtrusively was so complete and so personal, that it not only gave me tremendous peace of mind but also gave me a feeling of additional closeness to my dad and a feeling of satisfaction that I was contributing in a very significant way to his care and helping him remain independent in his own home. Technology actually can be warm and fuzzy, it seems.

It can also be a medical aid, remotely collecting vital-sign and health data and issuing medication or other reminders. Aerotel's MDKeeper, now in prototype mode, is a large watch-sized device that records pulse, oxygen saturation, and a one-lead EKG and transmits information continuously and wirelessly through cellular technology to a central monitoring station. The device even has a speaker to receive a call from central monitoring.

Another company, A&D Medical, offers a one-step auto-inflation blood-pressure monitor and a personal scale, both with wireless Bluetooth communication that can send real-time or batched-time/ date-stamped measurements to an access point. BeWell Mobile provides a technology platform and provides patient engagement software to incorporate self-monitoring of diabetes and asthma via cellular technology with the added emphasis on empowering patients. IBM in Zurich is close to releasing a pulse and blood-pressure wristband monitor—again like an oversized watch that transmits via Bluetooth technology. They have also focused on a pill box that similarly transmits to a central data point when a pill has been taken.

Other simpler and readily available assistive devices are 7-day, 28-compartment pill boxes with a small alarm clock and a 7-day memory that have a familiar look and do a lot while being low-tech and only costing $20 each. Vibrating-watch pill/blood-pressure-check reminders for the hearing impaired, and alarm watches with a dozen settings are available for $80 each. Posey makes a chair-seat monitor that triggers a small recorder that can remind you to use your walker or cane in a personalized way for $80. Tunstall in the UK carries a whole line of oversized switches/remotes/joysticks for those with arthritis to control their surroundings, and has also developed a variety of sensors to track your activity to gauge incipient change. They also have a fall sensor. Research continues in Ireland with a government/Intel collaboration called TRIL to focus on falls, dementia, and social interaction.

One of the most exciting pieces on the health-care side of our offerings will be working with eClinicalWorks, an incredibly progressive and robust electronic medical-records (EMR) company that has developed a portal through which patients can access all of their health data and participate more fully in their own health care. The company has partnered with Curas, an EMR mobile-device maker that connects physicians with the entire EMR system via cellular technology to allow comprehensive access to all patient information wherever the physician is and to manage the care from that point of access also. The costs are very affordable. The platform is exhaustive. My own medical office has used their EMR system for almost seven years, and it continues to grow in every right direction.

While there is a lot of "gee-whiz" to these gadgets, it is important to remember, the primary focus must not be medical. Secondly, these devices are merely tools to help one remain safely in one's own home.

The most important ingredient is the "people power" that this electronic social network can provide. Connected elders can take back their lives and restore meaning to them.

With these technology components added to personal in-home supportive care for a few hours per week, the Maine Approach offers an incredible package at a spectacular price. With daily review of the data, phone check-ins, community activity fulfillment, and varied volunteer opportunities included, not to mention being the family's first responder for trouble shooting, the Maine Approach offers comprehensive connections and peace of mind for all the family.

fourteen

The Maine Approach in Action

WE ARE BLAZING A NEW TRAIL HERE in Maine into an unknown frontier, and yet it is comfortingly familiar. The more chances we take, the more amazing and thrilling have been the discoveries. A few specific stories from the winter of 2009–10 will illustrate what I mean.

Almost Frozen—January 30, 2010

The focus of some of our important early work has been to use video technology to support elders in their homes and to keep them safe. One fortunate use of our video spot checking probably saved Elizabeth's life.

Elizabeth was a pleasantly forgetful, fiercely independent 98-year-old who lived alone in Alna, Maine. She never married and spent much of her life as a professional nanny for the well-to-do. She kept in touch with many now older adults that she helped raise long ago. Last fall with the help of her concerned neighbors, I arm-twisted her into accepting a video monitoring and elder-support package and installed a webcam in her living room with intermittent remote monitoring, mostly "to keep her concerned neighbors happy." She personally didn't see the need for any additional help.

One cold Friday night in January saw single-digit temperatures with strong winds. Saturday morning when our volunteer did his spot webcam checks, Elizabeth was sitting on her living room couch bundled up in her winter coat and blankets. Our team sprung into action. Our nurse manager and Elizabeth's "guardian angel," Carol, called Elizabeth's neighbor and personal advocate, Amy, who was busy serving breakfast at the Alna Store across the street. Amy and another store patron immediately went to Elizabeth's home and found her blue, shivering, and speaking incoherently. The house was ice cold.

Together, they scooped her up, and wrapped in blankets, carried her across the street and plunked her in front of the hot-air blower of the massive space heater in the front corner of the store. A couple of other restaurant patrons, with winter first-aid training, had just returned from winter camping, and took over rewarming her by rotating warmed blankets, and forcing her to sip sweetened hot tea. Elizabeth responded nicely.

Our team called Al, another nearby Maine Approach client, to ask if they could use his warm house for an unscheduled respite care. No problem. He has a spare first-floor bedroom and a sunny south-facing picture window, and he is home all day every day anyway.

Another staffer, Jen, was finishing up serving breakfast to another at-home member not too far away. Could she pick up Elizabeth shortly and bring her to Al's, check on him, take Elizabeth's temperature, tuck her in, and report back? No problem. Elizabeth's temperature was 92.7 almost two hours after being found! More tea, more blankets, a very warm house, a sunny window, regular temperature checks, and she was 97.6 in four hours. A high-tech emergency room could not have done this any faster.

Elizabeth napped in the sun while Al read the paper and puttered about. Amy from the Alna Store had now caught up with her work and brought them both a hot lunch, pushed more fluids, reassessed her neighbor and friend, and found her to be back to her baseline. Al was put in charge for the afternoon with Jen and Amy close by. There were remote webcam checks almost continuously, and a planned reassessment at supper. Some reading, some television, some small talk, a Saturday visit from one of Al's kids made for a busy but comfortable afternoon for both of them. Al very appropriately called Amy at the Alna Store when Elizabeth started getting a bit confused after sundown. He also ordered takeout for them both.

Elizabeth's take was "Why all the fuss?" She remembered shivering, but her memory loss precluded a more expansive account of the day. But she adamantly wanted to return home to sleep in her own bed. She got a profound positive emotional bounce from the attention and new community connections. The next week she continued to be more animated, more self-reliant, and more inquisitive about the local community than she had been in months.

Al's take: He got a lot more company than usual, welcomed the hustle and bustle, and felt good about being needed and useful. Which he truly was. Here was elder-to-elder volunteerism at its best.

By 9:00 PM, the furnace problem had been corrected. Elizabeth had inadvertently shut off the furnace emergency switch rather than the cellar light switch. The pipes were all checked for leaks by volunteers, and the Alna Store closed for the night. Amy and I reassessed Elizabeth, and Amy brought her back home with a few additional safeguards in place. The culprit furnace switch was now tightly duct-taped in the "on" position. Elizabeth was so buoyed by her good day that she coaxed Amy into staying for two hours longer to watch a movie with her on her favorite TV station, the Hallmark Channel.

My take: It was too close a call, but a job well done by all. No emergency room, no paramedics, no hospital bills. We had helped Elizabeth successfully within the constraints of her adamant wishes to stay at home. We would have been ill-equipped to handle a re-warming arrhythmia but other than that, I felt we had pushed the envelope, and had achieved an excellent outcome. A fragile but determined woman was still home living where she preferred to be.

The alternative scenario that could have ensued would have been an emergency room visit with a very frightened, demented woman struggling with a whole team of professional strangers as they asked her many questions that confused her. They would have wrapped her in an inflatable suit called a bear-hugger, placed BP/P/O$_2$ saturation monitor wires and self-inflating automatic cuff on her arm, with warmed, humidified oxygen tubing in her nose, an IV or two in her arms, a Foley catheter in her bladder irrigated with warm fluids. Then, most of the day later, she would have been admitted to a cardiac-monitored hospital bed to meet another team of caregivers with more questions that would confuse her.

A couple of days later, the hospital discharge planning team and physicians would have deemed her too weak and too fragile to go home. So after she had met the requisite three-hospital-night provision of Medicare to qualify for a rehab stay, she would have been moved to the skilled nursing facility by ambulance to meet another team of caregivers in a different room with a different routine.

With luck her hospital stay would not have been complicated by finding more issues to address. She would have avoided an ICU-provoked psychosis to medicate, or a bladder infection to treat. Then, a few weeks later, the skilled nursing social-service and physical-therapy teams may have found her still too fragile to live alone safely, and have recommended to her out-of-state distant relatives and her physician that she needed to reside in a long-term care facility for the rest of her life. How many would aggressively advocate for her to avoid this fate? What were the relative costs and personal satisfaction scores of these two scenarios?

Instead, more visits and respite daycare are in store for both Elizabeth and Al and the whole Maine Approach network. Temperature sensors are now incorporated into everyone's packages, and others will benefit from the feedback of these two isolated neighbors being introduced.

The Flannel Inn

Mother Nature forced us to improvise again later that winter. The story of the "Flannel Inn" taught us even more about Alzheimer's disease.

Thursday, February 25, 2010, saw wind gusts of 50–60 mph with heavy rain along the coast of Maine, and one to two feet of snow in the higher elevations. It was pretty nasty weather, even by Maine standards, and electrical power was out in much of the area. Yet 94-year-old Ed, who no longer drives at night, was still hoping he could go play cribbage in Wiscasset. Partly because after recently spending a month in the hospital and rehab facility recovering from a life-threatening pneumonia that many thought he might not survive, at some level he knew he should not squander any opportunity to enjoy life. On another level, after being a park warden on top of Mount Katahdin for much of his adult life, he may not have been bothered by a little wind. On still another level, his flexibility to roll with the punches life and Mother Nature threw his way may be why he has lived so long.

Ed is not careless. He also trusts and appreciates his Maine Approach support team to help him make the right decisions.

When I picked him up for his return trip home from cribbage, I commented on his use of his walking stick rather than the walker he was using two weeks ago. Vanity or improvement, I wondered. "Oh, I don't need the walker anymore anywhere, home or out. I even built a fire today in the woodstove to take the chill off." Which meant he had navigated the cellar stairs with some firewood. Impressive.

Somehow, his 120-pound frame avoided being blown over, he kept his narrow-brimmed hat on his head, and got himself into the car. On the way home, he guided me expertly through the low-lying water overflowing onto Bremen Road, and around the sink holes on his Cove Road. Then, with a spry step and a nonchalant wave, he disappeared through the garage and into his home. Good for you, Ed, I thought. It made me smile deep inside.

By 8:00 AM, Amy at the Alna Store wanted to bring 98-year-old Elizabeth—yes, Elizabeth again—who was without power, to 83-year-old Al's house a few miles away. Al's house had never even had the lights flicker in the fifteen years he had lived there. He must be on the trunk line for the electric grid for his area.

Charlie, another neighbor, called Al to see if there was room for Dorothy, the 90-year-old elder he cares for 24/7 in his own home as he was without electricity.

Bill and Anita from Jefferson were in the emergency department because Bill was short of breath and could not operate his nebulizer without electricity. He was too winded to get the generator started. When the hospitalist wanted to admit him, he declined, saying the Maine Approach network team would help. Sure enough, we found a neighbor, Kim, who brought them a meal, started a fire for them in their cellar woodstove, and even loaned and started a small generator to get them through the night. A few phone checks through the evening and the following morning confirmed that Bill's breathing was satisfactory, and they were warm.

By 1:30 PM, the power was back on at 96-year-old Helen's; 103-year-old John was okay; 88-year-old Rodney's generator was working well for him this time after we had overseen its tune-up last month; and 84-year-old Bobby and wife Sandy had a fire in the fireplace, an extra oxygen tank for the night, and a son borrowing a generator for the night. We continued to check the Maine Approach members.

The big dilemma was what to do about Stella? She was 90, without power, her son unavailable, and because of her moderate dementia, she rarely left her house. Our nurse Carol found Stella at home, covered in blankets, and still cold. In a matter-of-fact fashion, Carol told Stella she needed to leave with her now or she would die, and without protest, off they went to join the slumber party at Al's. This would be interesting: two quite demented 90-plus-year-olds in a strange house for a night or two or three, hosted by an 83-year-old man.

Elizabeth and Stella sat at the drop-leaf table in the living room while next-door neighbor Jen and I made up beds, and Amy from down the street, also without power, served them a hot meal. After they both denied being hungry, they consumed all their meatloaf, mashed potato, carrots, and even had room for pumpkin pie. Jen's daughter Michaela entertained them showing off her new pajamas, and Mike and Amy and their German shepherd rounded out the impromptu party.

The "girls" went to bed about 9:30 PM, had adapted very well to their new surroundings, and amazingly both found their own way unassisted to the spare bathroom during the night. When they woke up around 7:00 AM, they were a bit bewildered as to where they were, and who were these strangers, and how did they get there. It led to some lively explaining that they took in stride.

Stella was able to return home midmorning, but Elizabeth's power was out for another two nights. She managed uneventfully until then. Host Al actually enjoyed all the goings-on, and felt a little let down when the "Flannel Inn" closed down on Monday. I was as amazed as anyone.

If you had tried to tell me that you could take the very old, with severe dementia, and move them successfully to a new surrounding on the spur of the moment, and have such a stay go off without a hitch—I would not have believed it. It defies conventional wisdom. But it worked, surprisingly well. If only Gram could have been there, she would have loved it.

The most important ingredient to our success appeared to be a warm, gentle, reassuring manner without a lot of unnecessary explanation.

"Home Away From Home" Respite Care

Al would soon get another chance to play host. Ninety-two-year-old Elliott remodeled his home to have his daughter Jan live with him. After surviving lung cancer, and glaucoma, he moved quite slowly and carefully. Despite having worked as a maritime supervisor for a large oil company, his worldview was really quite restricted. And that was long ago. He is even more regimented in his behavior now. He can function quite nicely in his own home but needs reminders and company to eat very well or even use his breathing nebulizer.

If his daughter does not keep an eye on him, he is likely to poke around the yard and get into trouble with the riding lawnmower or some other project that is a little beyond his current mental and physical ability. But he is far from helpless.

As dedicated as Jan is to her father's care, she was exhausted. She also felt inhibited about taking care of her own needs, wanting to attend a week-long conference out of town. There were no respite care beds available at the local assisted-living facilities. As most of these facilities operate at full occupancy, rarely is there an available bed for short-term needs. Additionally, respite residents are a lot of work for a residential-care facility for a brief stay.

So we proposed a respite week for Elliot at Al's home while Jan took her course. By now, you might get the idea that Al lives in a single-story ranch with a spare bedroom. Al quickly welcomed the idea, and after the appropriate introductions on Monday morning, our nurse Carol brought Elliot over to Al's home. This was, to be honest, an experiment. Could one elder in our Maine Approach family be an effective volunteer host to another? And for an entire week? If so, the possibilities for using such home-away-from-home visits to meet the exploding respite care needs in our community and our country could be profound.

After weathering a few initial jitters, the arrangement flourished. Almost immediately, without any significant training or prepara- tion, Al became a capable caregiver. He was solicitous of Elliot's needs, making conversation, and adapting his daily routine some- what to accommodate him. They watched sports together with Al being challenged to explain some things to Elliot about the Red Sox' season. They listened to music, watched the honeybees buzz- ing around the cherry tree outside the kitchen window, and debated other tree types out in the distance.

At mealtime, supper was delivered for two rather than the usual one and a reminder given to both to take their medications. Al served dessert for both of them from the freezer and did the dishes. Elliot was provided with an emergency-response button, even though Al would have been comfortable summoning help by phone if needed. Our webcam video spot-checker was informed of the new arrival, and peeked in on both periodically to make sure all was going smoothly.

During Al's nighttime bathroom visit, and morning clean-up routine, it was heart-warming to capture him on video checking to see that Elliot was okay. Jen, the personal support attendant, who sees Al daily, arrived midmorning to help with breakfast, personal hygiene, and set up lunch for when they were hungry. Our Maine Approach volunteer phone captain called Al in the early afternoon to provide another personal reassurance and another personal touch.

Through the course of Al's typical week, updated regularly with his Maine Approach personal advocate, Elliott was treated to a couple of homemade meals delivered from the Alna Store, and a couple of meals out with Al's grandson Ben. By the time I took them both out to the annual Fisherman's Festival in Boothbay Harbor Saturday morning for a surreptitious debriefing, it was apparent that some quite profound transformations had taken place in that short week.

Elliott had dusted off some dormant social skills, and although still more inwardly focused than the average, he was again beginning to notice couples, children, dogs, cars, and fashion around him. He progressed before my eyes from bewilderment at the crowd to sharing his observations with us. He had changed his position sitting in the park or on the porch periodically so that he could people-watch better.

Al, for his part, became more independent. Struck by Elliot's physical and mental limitations, he worked harder to minimize his own. He took his own medications more often without cuing, did more dishes, made his own bed more often, even took out the trash to the garage. He was with a peer and also had newfound responsibilities. His own social skills and pride propelled him to perform respectably. As the week ended, Elliott packed up his things, received an L.L. Bean baseball cap from Al as a parting gift, and both agreed to see each other again. They may not become inseparable friends, but each profited handsomely from the arranged "sleepover."

What we learned was that elders are far more resilient than we give them credit for. They are also dramatically affected by the expectations others have of them, and how these expectations shape their daily lives. Let us first return to Al again to give a striking example of what I mean.

In September 2009, Al underwent spinal stenosis surgery, and went to the skilled nursing facility a few days afterward for reha-bilitation. He remained quite confused throughout his stay in the facility, although he did improve somewhat, the longer he had a set routine, and the more his health-care team avoided pain medication, bladder medications, and frequent nighttime interruptions.

He had bed and chair monitors attached so that he could not get up without staff notification. Meals were delivered on schedule, with the entire meal tray set up and food even unwrapped for him. He watched a lot of television but struggled with the remote control. What was on at the time, stayed on. He had his favorite daily news-paper, the *Boston Globe*, delivered by a family member, but he looked at it infrequently. Therapists came often for his sessions, and staff checked on him frequently. You would have thought the human interactions would have enlivened this man who lived alone, and genuinely enjoyed other people's company. Yet, slowly but surely, he became duller mentally, and took less initiative. A part of him liked being waited on. It was a lifelong familiar pattern for him. Within a few weeks, however, even though his restrictions had been loosened somewhat, we wondered whether he would be able to return home again. He had become so dependent on others for the simplest of daily activities. But he did not seem happy either.

The physical-therapy progress he made was terribly slow. He only walked when pushed. He scuffed his right foot occasionally but rather than a near fall, it appeared to produce a momentary loss of balance that he could easily and completely self-correct. He demon-strated to me again and again the ability to compensate adequately. His fall risk therefore seemed to me quite acceptable.

However, this environment was making him completely depen-dent. Clothes were washed and laid out for him. He dressed only when someone suggested it. He was encouraged to use the bath-room according to staff availability to assist him, not according to his own need. He did not even have to recognize hunger, and walk to the next room to eat. Food arrived automatically without any involvement on his part.

I had never appreciated what an important role recognizing hunger and acting upon that impulse plays in our activity of daily living. After six weeks, it seemed that the sooner he returned home, the better chance he would have to regain some of his independence.

His return home was planned for when a family member could stay with him the first few nights. He managed without incident. The Maine Approach webcams provided additional insights. Watching his activity remotely gave us a truer picture of his safety, unfiltered by trying to please a therapist. Seeing him navigate around obstacles in his home was very reassuring to us. However, watching him try to do everyday things alone with a walker was also instructive. Imagine getting around in the standard bathroom with a walker. Imagine how you would get clothes out of a bureau with a walker, or open the refrigerator door and access the shelves. Imagine how awkward it is to reach a tabletop lamp switch without readjusting your walker's position several times. It was quite clear that although walker use may be in the best interest of a nursing facility intent on demonstrating their commitment to fall-risk prevention, a walker in no way facilitates independence at home. In many ways, it invites disaster and contributes to many accidents.

Over the course of the next two weeks at home, Al made rapid progress. He slowly weaned himself from the walker. His best strengthening program was walking to the refrigerator and the bathroom many times a day. His mental agility improved as he had to think for himself most of the time. His Maine Approach helpers Carol and Jen did not cut him any slack. He was expected to do as much for himself as possible. In the skilled nursing unit he had been pampered, and it almost kept him there forever.

As alluded to earlier, the key was in providing Al not just with more or less stimulation, but the right stimulation. Wrong stimulation is just as counterproductive as isolation. It may not always be possible to know ahead of time what the right interplay is with any individual at any given time. But like most things, when it works, you know it when you see it, and you can derive great satisfaction from that encounter while the elder gets an amazingly long-lasting positive emotional bounce from that interaction.

Our voyage of rediscovery was forced upon us by the impossibility of serving our older friends and neighbors through a financially unsustainable institutional system. In a sense, this was fortunate, as it gave us the freedom to think creatively about what really matters to our elders and how much medical intervention they really require to be safe and secure.

• fifteen •

Early Successes and Tough Lessons

THIS CHAPTER INCLUDES MANY OF the case histories of the people who have been the brave pioneers that have embraced our vision. You have met some of them before. They have all helped refine our approach dramatically by sharing their lives with our staff, trusting us to care for them and do right by them. It is their faith and determination that has given substance to our vision.

While some of the earlier vignettes gave you the flavor of our elder cohort, the following summaries demonstrate how the more challenging situations can still be handled by the Maine Approach. If we can handle these tough scenarios, the Maine Approach can work for most elders in most communities.

The first person to showcase is our poster girl, 96-year-old Helen. Helen had been a patient of Full Circle Family Medicine for many years when she fell at home in autumn 2007 and landed in the hospital. She recovered at the long-term-care unit for a few months until she came to a crossroad. She qualified for permanent long-term care at the nursing facility according to the established assessment process in Maine but wanted to return home. She had lived in the same home on High Street since long before her husband died ten years earlier. That home contained the familiarity that she wanted for the rest of her life. She accepted the concerns of her daughter and me that returning home may not work. But she wanted to try. Helen had received very fine care at Cove's Edge Nursing Facility and had endeared herself to the staff, but she missed her neighbor, Kermit, who often brought her the morning newspaper and stayed for a cup of coffee and some conversation. She missed puttering around in the workshop attached to her home where her husband had done his photography work. Many of his tools of the trade were still there. She liked to sit in the front parlor in the afternoon sun, and stay there to read the paper, or sometimes later watch the evening news on television. She liked to eat when she was hungry. Her preferred meal was an English muffin with peanut butter. She did, however, often eat the Meals on Wheels offering if she knew the driver and if he stayed long enough to share some small talk.

With her daughter's blessing, I offered Helen the opportunity to return home with our fledgling remote-monitoring support program. She jumped at the chance. We installed motion sensors and a webcam, and every noon, her guardian angel, nurse Carol Richards, came over to fix her lunch. Helen ate better if Carol stayed with her, so Carol adjusted her schedule accordingly and did laundry, straightened up the house, and just chatted about life then and now. Helen shared stories and slowly got stronger. Despite our apprehension about her frailty, she lived two and a half years without an emergency-room visit. Carol adeptly identified problems early on. She took her out occasionally to the hair salon or just for lunch. We were able to monitor her remotely twenty-three hours a day and provided one hour a day of on-site personal care initially for about $700 per month rather than the $10,000 per month she was paying privately at the nursing home. Most importantly, she was happy. She continued to reaffirm that being in her own home was what she desired.

As she declined, she walked less, and spent more time in her bedroom. Still, she was surrounded by her familiar things. Our volunteers visited her more often, and she always rose to the occasion to charm them with her stories and her engaging manner. After we discovered with our motion sensors that she had fallen once, we installed a second camera in her bedroom. We were careful to position it to respect her privacy, while still capturing her in her danger zone between bed and bathroom. A few times, we identified a fall, and our tele-caregiver notified our designated responder.

She escaped injury every time. Once when no one else was available, I went to her rescue about 2:00 AM. When I got there, she nonchalantly greeted me warmly, and congratulated me on my good timing, as she indeed needed a little assistance. Our remote monitoring was so unobtrusive she continued to forget the camera was there. But she knew she was home, and steadfastly insisted this was where she wanted to be.

After two and a half years, she finally had an episode that required an emergency-room visit. She fell softly as usual, but in trying to get up, she pulled a TV tray down on top of her and got a small scalp laceration. No stitches were needed, but it sure bled a lot, causing our dedicated volunteer responder Marie to appropriately call for an ambulance. She lovingly reassured Helen during the transport and subsequent emergency-room visit. When the emergency physician and nurse tried to classify her as having an "unwitnessed fall," I proudly corrected them by Googling her remote camera from the emergency room and pulling up the entire sequence preceding her fall for their review. I showed the ambulance crew our arrival, their arrival, and the time-stamped images that nicely documented anything we wanted while also allowing us to annotate the snapshots. We had installed a night-vision camera in her bedroom for just such a purpose, as Helen kept turning off the night-light. Because she had such comprehensive home monitoring, she was able to return safely home after a very brief stay at the hospital.

Helen's story taught us other lessons. No longer was the adult daughter living nearby the family member who bore the entire burden of her mom's care. Another daughter of hers on the other side of the state, and a son in Colorado also visited the webcam daily, checked on their mom remotely, and provided some backup support that allayed some of their guilt about living so far away. They also derived great satisfaction from "seeing" their mother more regularly. Whenever family members needed that warm, personal "fix" of seeing a loved one in his or her own familiar surroundings, they could access the camera from their computer or cell phone anywhere in the world. Our tele-caregivers increased the frequency of their surveillance of Helen whenever any input triggered additional concern.

Our team was able to provide professional support in a low-keyed, very personal, noninstitutional manner that bridged many of the gaps between distant family members, a local working daughter, and a mother's decline that was often difficult for her family to watch. I believe being in her own home made these issues much easier for everyone to deal with.

This fragile, nursing-home-qualified, moderately demented woman was walker-dependent with end-stage arthritis in her hips, shoulders, and back. Since our approach kept her home without incident for almost three years, I believe we can address the needs of almost any elder. We saved her and her family alone over $250,000. And her personal satisfaction was infinitely better. Thank you, Helen, for trusting us. Your example will assist and inspire others.

Another early success was 87-year-old Maggie. She had moved from her beautiful home with its hilltop location surrounded by formal, terraced flower gardens. Her new residence at the upscale assisted-living village in Boothbay Harbor, Maine, was not working out so well. She "fired" one staff person after another, and her unmet care needs were driving her only son crazy. It sounded like a perfect situation for our new and personalized approach. With very little planning, we befriended her, installed a webcam, and provided an unflappable staff person, Carol, to see her briefly every day. In her own home, she quieted down nicely. Her home's open floor plan made monitoring easy. Learning her behavior remotely made tailoring her care and medication much easier. She prized her independence, especially her need to be in control. She wanted us in her home but on her terms. Our remote monitoring allowed that to happen unobtrusively, while still providing reassurance to Maggie and her family that we could respond to any difficulty in short order. Her son and daughter-in-law could see for themselves that she was managing acceptably. She functioned very well on her own for almost a year before she had a terminal medical event from which she succumbed after two weeks in the skilled facility.

One of the tough lessons Maggie's situation taught us was the delicate dance around the personal and legal responsibility for decision making in this elder cohort. Many elders, mentally competent in the eyes of the law, are unable to make all of the decisions necessary to preserve their independence. They need guidance and advocacy, and our fractured and widely dispersed families make that difficult. In Maggie's case, she had an involved son and daughter-in-law, but she did not want to cede authority to them. Third-party involvement from our staff and volunteers often got caught in the middle, generating no insurmountable problems, but alerting us to their dangers. Helping resolve family conflict has proven to go with the territory.

Next, Virginia represented another sturdy pioneering woman in our area. She convinced her husband to accept my recommendation to let some remote monitoring help them stay in their home together. Her husband, Doug, lived in the same house he had been born in. He had added a few electrical outlets, and a few rope pulleys to accommodate their advanced aging in a very cluttered home. He had a never-ending curiosity about new inventions, and loved to tinker to make do. After a lifetime of lobster fishing, he was no stranger to complex problem solving with what he had on hand. Despite an eighth-grade formal education, he had taught himself stock-market investing, and by being frugal, he had retired early and comfortably. He loved his various berry patches and fruit trees. He donated a large parcel to the local land conservation trust. He enjoyed and occasionally outfoxed the animals that interfered with his farm fruit. He babied his truck and tractor, and tried to tackle every repair project himself.

He took great delight in reminding his doctors that five and a half years earlier he had been given six months to live with his liver cancer. He took equal delight in managing his pills, adapting his diet to the shifting sands of his stomach and bowel conditions, and loved showing the doctors and nurses his latest modifications to colostomy care and edema management. He needed to be home to thrive and continue running his beloved farm. He also felt responsible for looking after Virginia, as they had been together for forty years.

With an emergency-response button, webcams, home visitors who were interested in his stories, and by allowing access to nurse or doctor advice without having to leave home, our package of services fit them nicely. These two 80-year-olds, who had met each other again later in life and had no children, were exceptionally well matched to look out for each other. For over a year, we enhanced their ability to stay at home, with our reassurance and our backup. This past March, acknowledging that he could no longer tend the wood-fired cookstove properly, could not care for his wife and farmhouse in his usual manner, and was done inventing new ways to address his care, he was ready to check out.

He did not want to burden Virginia by dying at home. So, even though we could have provided end-of-life care at home, he wanted to move to the skilled nursing unit to spare Virginia from dealing directly with that task. On a miserable, stormy night two weeks later, he died peacefully. Leave it to Doug to get Virginia back out on a miserable night. Now alone, his spouse of many years began the chore of learning to live without him. The new connections she had made with us would help nicely during this transition and afterwards. She hopes to volunteer to help others now that she does not have to worry about Doug.

Jim and Leona were another older couple intent on staying in their own home. Jim was 91, had fished his whole life, and had built a simple single-story retirement home overlooking his lobster dock and harbor. Despite his complaints of shortness of breath, and a little balance problem stemming from the large brain tumor removed more than a decade ago, he spent part of every day out in his workshop, solving some new problem around the home.

Jim's 88-year-old wife, Leona, had convinced her husband that trips to Florida for the winter now took too much out of them. They preferred Maine. Her memory was failing, and her husband needed to remind her about medications, meals, showering, and turning off the stove. But together they managed mostly. A dedicated granddaughter ran errands for them. A great grandson often stayed in the basement den.

Their concerned son, Dick, and his wife live in northern Vermont. They worry about Jim and Leona but can only visit periodically for a few days at a time. With access to our webcam service, they now "drop in" remotely on Mom and Dad whenever they have heightened concerns. Dick's sister, who spends most of the year in Panama, also comes and stays for a few months at a time. When she and her mom clash, our nurses, Carol and Janet, and PCA Jen will run interference and provide support within the complex family dynamic. We provide local backup and additional personal touches and four-times-a-day video spot checks to make sure all is stable.

When the Maine Approach nurse called one day to report that she suspected Leona had impetigo on her lower lip, she texted me a snapshot and we began an antibiotic promptly. Our approach avoids the challenges of getting her out to the doctor's office for a straightforward problem. Again, our role is to fit in, to add to the pieces the family has already figured out. Our primary mission is to help Jim and Leona achieve *their* goal of staying together in their own home.

Bobby and Sandy were another stalwart couple who helped us blaze this new trail. When Sandy faced yet another back surgery, and 80-year-old husband Bobby refused any temporary residential placement despite his failing health due to heart, lung, kidney, and brain issues, she turned to us to rescue them. We placed webcams in the kitchen and living room for four-times-a-day spot checks and committed to personal visits twice a day to cook meals, administer medications, do a little laundry and housekeeping, and provide some lighthearted social interaction.

We complemented the attention paid by Bobby's son and daughter who visited regularly but were unable to help their stepmother manage the home. We needed to make sure Bobby and Sandy were equally comfortable with our people and our approach. I trust that it is not too sexist to observe that it is often not an easy task to step onto another woman's turf, regardless of her age, and provide the needed support without upstaging her, changing the rules and roles in the home, and making her feel unnecessary. She continues to need purpose. So even when Sandy returned home from her surgery and rehab stay, quite weak and wearing a full-trunk, wraparound plastic molded body brace, she tried to do some laundry and make some meals. We had to be respectful of her needs and limitations while being sensitive to her emotions as well.

A few times, I had to fill in for staff because of illness or vacation. The opportunities that presented themselves sitting at the breakfast counter with Bobby on New Year's morning, or visiting with Sandy in the evening while she reminisced about going to country dances with Bobby, were magical moments. The insights into their lives and what mattered were priceless. Bobby was truly very easy to care for. He accepted things as they were, had realistic expectations, and appreciated what others did for him. He started from the premise that he had lived a good life. Having been a farmer during his working years, he accepted death as the natural order of things. He never lost the twinkle in his bright blue eyes or the easy smile that punctuated a good story told. He loved sitting in his easy chair looking over the open fields sloping toward Damariscotta Lake. He did not begrudge watching someone else mow the lawn now, though he enjoyed it immensely when he could still drive the tractor. He loved watching golf on TV, and reflected on the rounds of golf he played after taking up the sport very late in life. For an extra year, we helped his wife keep him home and content.

Bobby, like Doug, did not want to die at home, even though he loved it there. He knew Sandy would live there after his death. He wanted her to be able to remember their good times unencumbered by perhaps too vivid a picture of his last few days. So, a few days before his eighty-third birthday, he agreed to come into the hospital to see if we could fine-tune any of his medical conditions. When it proved impossible, he died peacefully, with no regrets, on his birthday.

The groundwork we laid with his wife Sandy allowed us to continue to help her through the transition from missing Bobby to starting to figure out life after him. Without our nurse, her friend Carol, I doubt she would have handled her husband's death nearly so well. The hardest part is not necessarily getting through the funeral and the immediate aftermath. It is often the weeks and months later on when life may have returned to normal for family and friends, but still difficult for the surviving spouse who is trying to discover what the future holds for her. It is in this new territory that our novel approach really excels.

Again, it is very much our attitude, not the technology, that distinguishes the Maine Approach from the rest of the health-care landscape. After Bobby's return home from a previous hospitalization, his insurance benefits provided him with home health services. His well-meaning but off-base home health nurse arrived and began to clean out the cupboards and refrigerator to eliminate any foods containing salt, which were off limits because of his heart condition. His discharge diagnosis drove her subsequent behavior, not the big picture of his limited life expectancy, and certainly not of his quality of life. Neither he nor his wife were included in any discussion of the pros and cons of his care or even given other options.

They were instructed, however, to place a large orange magnetic emblem on their refrigerator so the rest of the home health team including the ambulance crew (in case they were called) would know he did not want to be resuscitated. So the convenience of the health-care team trumped the sensibility of husband and wife who must live with a glaring reminder of his being on borrowed time whenever they open their refrigerator. How absurd!

Steve was another member whose complex interpersonal life challenged the entire local medical world. He was 88 years old and living as a recluse in southern Maine. His estranged wife, Marty, approached us about bringing him back to her home on the lake for end-of-life care. They had gone their separate ways ten years ago but had never formally divorced. Despite their often stormy relationship, she wanted to do whatever she could to help now. He was calling her daily, often in the middle of the night, seeking help. Her friends suggested she contact us. We met several times over a month as Marty struggled with difficult choices. His three children from his previous marriage had had little contact with him for years, and did not get along with her very well. Steve was almost paranoid about switching doctors. Given his complex medical profile of bladder, prostate and kidney cancers, insulin-dependent diabetes, heart disease, weight loss, weakness, dementia, and an ever-expanding painful mass in his abdomen, the idea of moving him to the home of his nonmedical wife to oversee his care seemed crazy at best, and likely downright impossible.

With our encouragement, they tried a new residential hospice house. The medications got administered very reliably, but the phone calls did not stop. The complex unresolved personal issues between Steve, Marty, and the adult children escalated. Marty and our nurse Carol brought Steve to Newcastle. Our Maine Approach team entered this minefield with great apprehension but determined to try to answer a sincere request for help from a member of our community.

The first week saw an extraordinary transformation, though it taxed our people resources to the max. Separating out physical from emotional pain, working with his temper and his dementia, adjusting pain medication and diabetes medication, cutting curled-under toenails, removing earwax, setting up a daily routine for meals, toileting, other activities, and visitors were enormous challenges. Marty had lived alone in her immaculate, stunning, lakeside home for years. Oriental rugs and antique furniture clashed with uncooperative bodily functions.

By the end of the week, Steve was walking with standby assistance to the sunny porch for a midday meal or to meet a friend or relative. In the evening, Marty and Steve usually watched the news and often an old movie. We attempted to give Marty only the responsibility that she wanted and could handle. What she had signed on for was very tough. But with nurse Carol's guidance and patience, some semblance of a routine developed.

At times extraordinary circumstances called for extraordinary measures. Steve's dementia combined with his prior take-charge personality to produce a tragic yet comical situation a couple of months before he died. He had become distressed that the home-health hospice team visiting him was holding him hostage in this home. He wanted out. So despite his faltering gait, his delusional thinking, and chronic pain from his cancer, he left the house, walked down the driveway, and was standing in the middle of the road. He refused the attempts of his wife and his caregivers to coax him to come inside.

A panicked call to Carol saved the day. She arrived in our company Dodge Caravan, promptly acknowledged his distress, and asked him what he wanted to do? He replied that he needed the police. So she got him easily into the van under the pretext of addressing his expressed wish. Once he was seated, she phoned her husband at work to ask a favor. Would he impersonate a police officer for a few minutes? She then got into the van, explained to Steve what she would do for him, and with his permission she called the "police-man" on his behalf. She then handed the cell phone to Steve. He vented his concerns about the outrageous behavior going on at his home. "Officer" Richards heard him out, dutifully took down the details of his complaint, repeating them back to Steve, and assured him he would file a full report. Meanwhile, Carol cleared out the personnel that had incited Steve's wrath. Crisis addressed, Steve then calmly returned to the house. He never mentioned that episode again. Was this benign deception ethically sound? It's hard to say, but thinking outside the box diffused a potentially ugly and escalating situation.

To reiterate, the Maine Approach attitude already exists in just about everyone and can be developed and nurtured. We tap into the same natural talents of many who enter health care as a career, desiring to be of service. Unfortunately, in the current training of most health-care workers, the focus is on protocol, cookbook solutions, and using medications, law enforcement, and limited behavioral tools to manage unruly elder patients. The Maine Approach solution tries to understand the angst of even the most confused elder mind, and approach the situation uniquely. These elders are often wound very differently than other younger patients.

More generally, the Maine Approach means connecting with the individual. Rather than heed the colder, professional advice to "not get too involved" with the patient's plight, we stick our necks out. We seek to take the time and interest to advocate for each individual as best as we are able from their perspective. This requires different skills, not commonly taught in health-care training today but definitely teachable, and recognizable. We suspect that these traits are drummed out of many caregivers. It remains to be seen whether our assumptions are true that these characteristics can be re-instilled with training and workshops.

In any case, Steve remained at his wife's home for three months, punctuated by many poignant moments with family and friends. By no means did all of the emotional baggage of decades melt away. But together we accomplished much that many would have considered impossible. Steve died peacefully with his dignity intact. His story once again affirmed our way of doing things and that complex situations can be handled by the Maine Approach.

Rodney was another of our refugees from the assisted-living world. Almost 90, he used a walker, living independently in his own home for several years after his wife's death. He had also managed to learn to manage his colostomy care for more than a decade. He first sought our help a couple of years ago when a friend told him how we had helped him return home from an assisted-living facility. Rodney had reluctantly agreed to move into the assisted-living facility at his daughter's insistence a couple of months earlier. He sarcastically referred to it as "the Big House" and desperately wanted to be home with his two long-haired cats, and his books, in the home designed and built under his supervision.

In his own home, he knew where the open spaces were where he needed his walker. He also knew where he could "furniture walk" without it. At home, he remained engaged in conversations with his longtime housekeeper and errand person, Judy, who also brought back for him memories of his connections to his only son who was now deceased. Our staff came twice a day to fix meals and provide companionship. Webcam monitoring and motion sensors alerted other tele-caregivers about any potential problem. There was more detailed reporting available about him at home than exists in many expensive nursing homes.

Friends and occasional family visited when they could. Every inch of his home contained a chapter of memories about some part of his life. He maintained personal control of the parts of his day-to-day life he could still manage, and most of those around him who were still important in his life ceded this territory to him whenever possible. It was a complicated package but it worked well. The Maine Approach by design worked around these pieces. Our staff made suggestions. Our volunteers seized the opportunities he presented for a trip to a town festival, to have someone play his piano, to go for a ride to the farmers' market, to go to sit at a picnic table by the lake, to organize visits from other neighbors and friends of his, or to play cribbage regularly with another volunteer member.

Then a bacterial infection from bladder to bloodstream landed him in the hospital. He had a resistant organism, and some physicians doubted he would survive very long off the antibiotics. So, he headed over to the skilled nursing facility for a protracted antibiotic course.

Further decline set in, and a couple of months later, off antibiotics, and remaining urinary-tract symptom-free, he actually faced far bigger challenges. He hoped he would not survive long-term in a place he did not want to be. We were bucking the conventional wisdom to suggest he could return home. Health-care facility staff had convinced his family and his physician that there was no way Rodney could live safely at home any longer. Although he repeatedly said that he wanted to return home, he was too confused much of the time to advocate for that position. In addition, his insurance paid for residential care but not for at-home care, so returning home would also put him at a financial disadvantage, especially if he required a significant amount of care.

Some friends, relatively unfamiliar with all the details outlined above, expressed the sentiment that he was better off in the institutional setting than being alone at home. Others saw him in this sterile setting and sensed a profound sadness in the man. Despite a lot of people around him, in the halls, in the dining room, he seemed very alone. There was not enough to do. There was not enough of the right things to do. The sparkle was going out of his eyes. He was moved from the skilled rehab unit to the long-term-care unit, and a few weeks later, he suddenly ran a fever, developed an abdominal pain, received some morphine for comfort, and died the next day. I wish we had had another opportunity to try to make a stay back home work for him. He was such a sweet man, a perfect gentleman.

Ethel first came to us as a video-calling companion for Barbara. As residents of two separate ElderCare Network homes fifteen miles apart, they had never met each other. Ethel had been a home health aide prior to having a major stroke in her early sixties. She constantly struggled with finding the words to express her thoughts, but had no deficits in her arms or her legs. She loved to dance. Moreover, she could still create fine poetry and paint delightful watercolors with the intact right side of her brain. She just could not read her poetry aloud because of damage to her speech center. Being relatively young, and very energetic, she did not fit in well with many assisted-living home residents. As she was single with two out-of-state sons with families of their own, her inability to live independently left her no other option.

Barbara was a verbal firecracker in a body racked by emphysema and diabetes. She was in her mid-seventies and dependent on an oxygen tube at all times. Yet she was outgoing, and very mobile within the confines of her assisted-living home. She loved to knit and was very proficient at it. But she irritated the other residents by trying to take over and being bossy. She was a good match for Ethel. So we introduced them as video buddies and a beautiful thing happened. Barbara gushed over Ethel's work, proudly displaying it to anyone she ran into, and becoming her mouthpiece. Ethel embraced their friendship, and enthusiastically returned Barbara's warmth, quite desperate for more human interaction.

However, the caregivers at both homes underappreciated the importance of their connection. Barbara's demands for primary control of the living-room computer riled other residents, and attempted peacemaking by the staff was poorly handled. In the other home, Ethel's neediness for attention and activity accelerated beyond the capacity of the small staff, and they wouldn't embrace the computer connection. Ethel needed them to stretch for her and they did not. Something as simple as bringing Ethel to town on errands regularly would have helped. Another resident made fun of her language difficulties, bringing out an ugly side of human behavior at any level: the need for a pecking order. Over time, outings with volunteers were not frequent enough, and Ethel became unhappy.

A change was needed. But the change arranged by her legal advocate was to a dementia unit nearby. At first, Ethel was happier. The move brought new faces, new attention, and interestingly, a new people connection. She attached herself to a frail older female resident, and began helping her at mealtime. In short order, she had resurrected her old nursing-assistant skills, and relished the opportunity to be of service. The honeymoon period ended when the older resident was transferred to another nursing facility for higher needs people.

Now Ethel really began to struggle. She was surrounded by many souls with dementia in a locked unit with very little room to walk. There were not enough activities; or more precisely, not enough of the right activities. Ethel loved dance. When we took her to interpretive dance performances, or line dancing, or rock and roll, she was always the last one off the dance floor at the end of the night. When she attended choral groups, she wanted to be in every number.

When she was at an art class, they always ended too soon. She was starved for activities, and now she felt like a prisoner in a strange world. She became more frustrated and more desperate. With her language disorder, she had a hard time expressing her needs, and created more hardship for herself and others trying to understand her. Ethel's dilemma again symbolized the need not just for more or less stimulation. She needed the right stimulation.

Sarah lives in another assisted-living facility, and her story again epitomizes the difficulty of trying to find any good residential option for many older individuals. Originally from the Midwest, she raised four children and worked outside the home in public relations. After her divorce, circumstances surrounding a few less than ideal personal relationships alerted her children to her declining cognitive and decision-making capacity. She spent several years living with her supportive and attentive children until their personal and professional lives hampered the lives and relationships of all concerned. The family turned to assisted living hoping for more companionship and activity for their mom. Still only in her late sixties, Sarah was of a different generation than many of her housemates. A couple of volunteers greatly enriched Sarah's world with music and dance outside of the facility. Unfortunately, the facility's robust activity schedule ends in the late afternoon, and leaves long evenings empty for someone of Sarah's age and energy. The primary focus of the assisted-living home has historically been catering to older individuals who often call it a day after supper. Her situation called for a fresh look at their offerings.

Sarah's insights have pointed out other important shortcomings in our institutional approach to elder housing. Shortly after her arrival, she became very close to another resident who lived down the hall from her. They ate together at mealtime, and attended group activities together. They often visited each other in the slow times after supper. Then one morning her new acquaintance was not there.

When Sarah inquired of her whereabouts from the staff, they informed her that privacy rules prevented them from telling her where her friend was or what had happened to her. Talk about draconian measures! Human decency requires the staff and administration to show more creative sensitivity to those individuals who call their facility home. We are not talking about gossip. We are not talking about divulging intimate details of someone's life. We are simply talking about modest information that will allay an individual's fears, and let friends continue to reach out to one another.

The health-care world has been gripped by a kind of HIPPA paranoia that has spawned some insane interpretations of privacy protection. For example, when you call or visit the hospital nurses' station, it is rare that anyone will tell you if your friend has been transferred to the tertiary-care hospital, to the adjacent rehab facility, gone home, or even died. My wife volunteers often at various assisted-living facilities in our area, and has been regularly deprived of any information as to the whereabouts of her art students when they do not show up at class. No matter where one lives, the medicolegal climate must allow some common sense.

On a much less serious note, Sarah also reported to me how comical it is for her to get a glass of wine while she resides at the assisted-living facility. Residents are not allowed to keep alcohol in their rooms for fear of an adverse interaction with medications. So Sarah must approach the nurses' station and ask who is bartending this evening. They then pour her a glass of wine and away she goes.

Neal and Ginny are another local couple whose rich former lives prepared them nicely for a role in the Maine Approach. Their daughters Linda and Karen are very committed to their parents' welfare. When Linda first approached us, her parents had already decided to try the very nice Chase Point Assisted-Living Facility built and run on the local hospital campus by Miles HealthCare. After only a month there, they were ready to move back home. Being such social people, they enjoyed the staff and the other residents. But as Neal simply put it, "It wasn't home. It wasn't our home." They missed their dog, their cat, and their well-established routine in their own home. Chase Point was a nice vacation, and did allay many of Neal's worries about adequately attending to his wife's mental decline. He knew he needed more help, but wasn't there a better way? With our help, they not only had remote video monitoring, but the personal-care assistance to make meals, run errands, attend doctor's appointments when their daughters were unavailable or at work.

We filled in around the rest of the family, varying the support week to week. Our staff was able to nudge Ginny and Neal to do a little more for themselves. Their care needs reduced over the first year of our involvement, contrary to the typical scenario. Our philosophy could push Neal to do more for himself while also allaying his fears of being unable to leave Ginny alone. We could enable him to still be somewhat involved in the community organizations that were so important to him. We could enlist a volunteer who shared Ginny's passion for doll making to visit regularly. Respite day care will likely be her next need.

The take-home message is that the Maine Approach has proven it is robust enough to address comprehensively the complex needs of frail elders. A bona fide alternative to the residential-care facility now exists. Remote monitoring, interactive technology, a sprinkling of high-quality professional staff, and a few dedicated personal-support staff can handle complex elder members' needs in their own homes at 10 percent of the cost of existing residential-care options.

sixteen

The Dignity of Risk

WHENEVER I ENGAGE IN A DETAILED discussion about our core mission of helping elders remain in their own homes, invariably the conversation turns to liability. "Aren't you afraid of getting sued if something bad happened while you were involved in an elder's care at home?" "How can you prevent something untoward from occurring?" Maybe my family-practice medical training has made me more comfortable with uncertainty. Perhaps I am too laid-back about our litigation-obsessed and risk-averse society. In any case, I freely accept that any endeavor entails risk and the certainty that navigating the complex terrain of aging will regularly produce unexpected twists and turns.

"The dignity of risk" is a phrase that grew out of the experience of those who promoted the deinstitutionalization of the developmentally disabled during the 1970s. That entire cohort was deemed incapable of living on its own in the community. Many were thereby deprived of experiencing the richness of the full human experience. That richness included the opportunity to succeed or fail, and the opportunity to learn from that experience.

The whole idea of "the dignity of risk" resonates nicely with me as our Full Circle America approach tries hard to push the medical establishment and adult children to empower elders to continue to live independently, and thus to live their lives to the fullest for as long as they live. Despite limitations acquired over a lifetime, and varying enormously in severity, our elders deserve the opportunity to continue to make the daily decisions, big or small, that are part of daily living.

All too often, when an adult son or daughter visits an aging parent, one notices something mental or physical that the parent does that is less than ideal. Rather than accept such behavior as an expected consequence of aging, they all too often seek to remedy that behavior or even conclude that its existence is reason enough to deny that individual's ongoing right to live independently. Perhaps we have all grown so accustomed to our parents having all the answers that we cannot accept that they no longer possess that all-knowing capacity with which we long credited them.

Understandably it saddens us to see the individuals that nurtured us start losing their abilities. We feel a personal sense of loss as we grieve for no longer having their wisdom to bail us out. We are undeniably now responsible for some decisions we often feel totally unprepared to make. Perhaps we do not fully grasp the magnitude of forcing an older individual out of his or her home. In our ignorance, we often incorrectly assume that additional office visits, more medications, more therapies, or even a move to a residential-care facility will restore Mom or Dad to their prior position in our lives. Like other previous transitions in our relationships with our parents, this one especially requires some getting used to.

If I had lived in the same home for fifty or sixty years, how traumatic would it be to move? If I knew every creak in the floor, every threshold, and where every piece of furniture was placed, even in the dark, how unsettling would it be to move to completely new surroundings? If I had rooms of memorabilia that represented decades of experiences, and gave witness to the fact that I had lived a rich life and had been a meaningful contributor to the world around me, what have I lost when I am moved to a relatively sterile living unit and do not have those hundreds of smells, nooks, and crannies to jog my memory? How do I know who I am when I am reduced to a few mementos that are supposed to be representative of a lifetime?

We must get away from our risk-averse stance where older individuals are segregated from the rest of the community, and severely limited in their living arrangements in order to improve compliance with medication usage, and theoretically improve their safety. What will we accept in return for not missing a dose of medicine? We adult sons and daughters have been brainwashed into believing that our parents are no longer able to live independently, and that we are not expert enough to help them navigate daily living. Too many of our parents are either meekly acquiescing to the choices we made on their behalf or are equally unable to assess the full future consequences of these decisions.

When we do get involved and make a series of sensible choices with them on their behalf, we are often surprised to find that something that we did not expect happens. Either a component works enormously better than we could have possibly anticipated, or an equally reasoned choice turns out to be a very bad idea. That is life. And whichever outcome occurs allows us to shape subsequent choices with the benefit of that previous experience.

To me that is the meaning of the dignity of risk. We do not have the option of saying we will only embrace a course of action if it is guaranteed to succeed. Like many challenges we faced raising our own children, this time of life requires making the best choice with the information you have at hand, and moving forward. As others who navigated similar paths in other fields have noted in many ways, we will learn from the choices we make, and we need to accept that.

It's a commonplace that every opportunity for growth carries with it the possibility of failure. Accompanying every endeavor is an element of risk. If growth truly implies a chance for improvement, then it must also carry with it the chance that there will be no change, no improvement, or even failure. When a person's environment is overprotected in such a manner that there is little or no chance for failure, then in reality there is also little or no chance for real or significant success. To deprive someone of the opportunity for significant achievement because of an associated element of risk is to deprive them of their potential for growth.

This brings me to a few personal stories about elders that illustrate where we often go wrong. Many years ago, I made a 95-year-old man cry. Stanley had been driving a car since the first horseless carriages arrived in South Bristol in the early 1900s. He'd never had an accident, and now as his family doctor, at the behest of his son and neighbors, I was taking his license away. "But I only drive a few miles," he protested. Within a short period of time, he began to lose weight (due in part to not getting to the area lunch counter), and to neglect his own self-care more obviously (having given up on life in many ways). After a brief hospital stay, a move to a nursing home was advised. There he sat more than twenty miles from everything he valued.

One afternoon, perhaps out of guilt, while making rounds at his facility, I asked him if he wanted to go see his hometown's junior high basketball team play my son's team at the Great Salt Bay School. There was no hesitation on his part, and with a wheelchair and my signature, away we went past some disbelieving staff into the December darkness. I had not thought through what we were going to do, but I was confident we could figure it out. Getting Stanley into and out of my sedan was the hardest part. Rolling him into the gym and negotiating the bleachers was equally challenging. But the look on his face, and the size of his eyeballs, as we watched the game transcended any logistical problems. Watching for his great-grandnephew was completely engrossing. After the game, we used the opportunity to take a brief tour of downtown Christmas decorations, and then returned to the nursing home. For a few hours, he was reconnected to the rest of the community. He had stories to tell for the rest of his life. Could something unexpected have happened? Absolutely. Would I take such a chance again? Without a doubt.

Another afternoon, my wife volunteered me to take five elder women to the Lincoln County Community Theater for a Sunday matinee of the musical *Annie*. At that time, the theater lacked an elevator, and two stories of steep stairs brought you to the seating level. I thought that part would tax us the most. I had not anticipated getting them in and out of the ladies' room. With a little luck, and with the help of a few female theatergoers, we made it through just fine.

One of my guests was Marion. I probably have more "Marion stories" than those of any other patient. Several years earlier, she had interrupted me one afternoon while I was seeing patients to let me know her refrigerator had recently died. The Sears delivery man was at her home with a new one offering her one-, two-, and three-year warranties. Being the frugal independent woman she always was, she did not want to purchase a longer warranty than I thought she would live to enjoy!

Another time, she confessed that even though she had ghostwritten murder mysteries, it made her queasy to learn to take her own pulse to monitor her atrial fibrillation. Later that admission, when we gave her transient sedation to electrically cardiovert her heart's electrical system back to normal sinus rhythm, she opined that she was having the most delightful sleep and thought she must be in heaven, until she opened her eyes and saw me. She often commented that she had been fine until she met me, neglecting to add that we had met in the intensive care unit.

Still another time, determined to enjoy the view of Damariscotta Lake from our deck, she hiked up her skirt, and crawled up the cottage stairs on all fours. Her arthritic knees would not deter this 90-year-old. She had a delightful afternoon.

Now back to the theater. After the performance, I asked Marion and my other guests to remain seated until I could bring the van to the theater door. Then I hustled to get the car, but not fast enough. Upon my return, Marion had tried to go down the steep stairs by herself and fallen. She was sideways, halfway down the stairwell, with one shoe on a higher stair, and a cane down below. Although on blood thinners and somehow unhurt, she was mortified that her wig had fallen off and people would see her bald head! I was grateful that no major disaster had resulted. Marion accepted risk, embraced life fully, and hardly ever said no to anyone offering her the opportunity to have some fun. She stubbornly remained in her own home until the last year of her life at age 94. She was trying to teach me about measured risk. Furthermore, she knew a lot about having proper priorities in her life. She was a gift to those that knew her.

Several years later, my wife invited many of the Hodgdon Green assisted-living home residents to a summer dance party at our barn. To our delight, up drove Gayle Yost, clinical-nurse coordinator, with the facility van filled with seven residents. Gayle was not intimidated by bringing frail residents out for an adventure on her own time on a Saturday afternoon. They were treated to Esther Mariani playing her electric guitar and singing songs from the Beatles to Tori Amos, a glass of wine or two, and a private belly-dance exhibition by Natifa Sakti. A couple of residents danced regularly on the dance floor, and everyone tapped their feet to the beat. They had a ball. Despite varying degrees of memory impairment, the specifics of that event were retold for weeks. Lack of staff, limited resident mobility, and a porta-potty made for some interesting moments that only embellished the event. Being risk averse would have deprived many of a very special afternoon.

The most ambitious undertaking was on the Fourth of July, when much of Lincoln County turns out at Damariscotta's waterside parking lot downtown behind Main Street stores for festivities and fireworks. Rock and roll bands play from flatbed trailers, Boy Scouts sell hotdogs and burgers, while community raffles, pizza slices, ice cream, fluorescent necklaces, babies in strollers, pre-teens evading their parents, adolescents furtively meeting forbidden friends fill your senses. It is an event, a mix of chaos and fun, that is unpredictable at best. Into this tightly packed sea of humanity, bordered by rocky coast, tidal water, cars, and pedestrian traffic, the town adds a fabulous fireworks display. After dark, from a marshy point just across the water, a barrage of light, noise, and smoke explodes over the heads of the crowd. No doubt many town departments and agencies have entertained many "what-ifs" in preparation for this annual event. Yet no concern trumps the intangibles of fun, community spirit, the excitement of this human experience with all its attendant unknowns. Measured risks were taken all around the event. It was the perfect location for concept of the dignity of risk to be personified by an intrepid group of elders.

Last year, into this atmosphere, from the alley beside the Colby & Gale gas station, with the setting sun at their backs, appeared a parade of rolling walkers and wheelchairs, a cavalcade of frail elders from Hodgdon Green's assisted-living home. Many who could not come loaned their walkers with fold-down seats to others for the long hike downtown. With caregivers Angela, Pat, and Janet bravely handling the troops, within minutes this unlikely contingent was incorporated into the crowd and activities. It takes courage to take those first steps, and it means taking some risks. Who would want to miss this marvelous scene? Hopefully they will be regulars at the event.

On that July evening, Jolan and Kathryn, Gerry and Freddie, Henry and Ken were all coconspirators in shaking us up a little. The night air was perfect. The sounds and sights and smells were unique to that one day. Everything was just right until the crowd began to disperse right after the fireworks grand finale. Dark now and approaching 10:00 PM, it was time for that uphill climb back to Hodgdon Green: one-half mile of dark, sometimes uneven, sidewalks, street crossings, and exuberant youth pushing through the crowd. All this added to the stuff of walkers and wheelchairs, tired limbs and minds. I expected some impatience. To my surprise, the residents did not complain. They had big smiles and more than adequate energy. Somehow, Betty did not tip over taking her motorized wheelchair over the Church Street curb, Henry did not have chest pain on the uphill in front of the bank, and Gerry did not fall down in the middle of Main Street. I did not run over any toes maneuvering the wheelchair through the crowd. As everyone settled in for ice cream back at Hodgdon Green, it was a great feeling to have had such a fine time together. It became one of those memories to cherish for a long time.

There was significant liability exposure for all involved in each of the activities just described. There is also significant liability in every more mundane moment in the daily lives of many of these very same people. A trip to the bathroom or to the kitchen can occasionally produce a dangerous fall. That is life. That is the reality our elders live with every day. Most will not shrink away from fully engaging in daily life unless we instill fear in them. It is the rest of us that must face the challenges that an elder's way of life poses for us.

Once again, perspective gained from the developmentally disabled community can enlighten us. The following questions were adapted from *Changing Expectations/Planning for the Future: A Parent Advocacy Manual* by Dorothy Sauber. They were framed by a father whose son was in a supported work program for the developmentally disabled in Richmond, Virginia. His father offered the following observations: What if you never got to make a mistake? What if your money was always kept for you? What if you were no longer given a chance to do well at something? What if you were always treated like a child? What if your only chance to be with people different from you was with your own family? What if any job you did was not useful but just busy work? What if you never got to make a decision? What if the only risky thing you could do was to act out or be difficult? What if you could not go outside because the last time you went, you fell down or you got lost? What if you took the wrong bus once and now you cannot take another one? What if you got into trouble once and now they restrict your activity because they always remember your "trouble"? What if you had no privacy? What if you could do part of the grocery shopping but were not allowed to do any because you were not able to do all of the shopping? What if you spent three hours every day just waiting? What if you never got a chance again because you are old?[1]

These observations pertain equally well to many elders I see being patronized by well-meaning family and caregivers. Another champion for the developmentally disabled, noted author Robert Perske, said it a little differently but with equal power in *Hope for the Families*.

> Overprotection may appear on the surface to be kind,
> but it can be really evil. An oversupply can smother

people emotionally, squeeze the life out of their hopes and expectations, and strip them of their dignity. Overprotection can keep people from becoming all they could become. Many of our best achievements came the hard way: We took risks, fell flat, suffered, picked ourselves up, and tried again. Sometimes we made it and sometimes we did not. Even so, we were given the chance to try. Persons with special needs need these chances, too.

Of course, we are talking about prudent risks. People should not be expected to blindly face challenges that, without a doubt, will explode in their faces. Knowing which chances are prudent and which are not—this is a new skill that needs to be acquired. On the other hand, a risk is really only when it is not known beforehand whether a person can succeed. . . .

In the past, we found clever ways to build avoidance of risk into the lives of persons living with disabilities. Now we must work equally hard to help find the proper amount of risk these people have the right to take. We have learned that there can be healthy development in risk taking . . . and there can be crippling indignity in safety![2]

Several years ago, John, a widower and retired architect, was trying very hard to live independently in an apartment in Damariscotta. On his bucket list was a lifelong desire to travel across Canada by rail. He wanted to do this by himself, and repeatedly affirmed that he knew the risks and wanted to take them. Having watched him survive a couple of strokes with only a little impairment of thinking and balance, his family was on the fence about accepting his decision. Yet, over months, his children became more comfortable with their own fears and eventually, John went. He survived. He did get lost a few times as best as anyone could ascertain. He met strangers who helped him. He returned content and fulfilled. It was courageous on everyone's part to let him go. It was a tribute to the respect with which his children always treated him that such a journey could be entertained and executed. It truly represented the dignity of risk for John.

Chris Lyons, a nationally recognized attorney specializing in the defense of community service providers, likes to illustrate the importance of building the dignity of risk into the lives of people with disabilities.

> Imagine . . . you wanted to go across the street from where you live to the corner store to get some ice cream. And in order to do that I had to go with you. And I had to decide when we went. And I had to decide how we went. And I had to decide what you did when you were there. . . . How would that make you feel as an individual? . . .
>
> Well let's change it a little bit. . . . I don't have to go with you across the street, but you do have to come to me to cross the street. And you have to ask me for permission to cross the street and I have to annually check you for "street crossedness.". . .
>
> Well, now I'm going by myself, so I feel a little bit better and it's a little bit more meaningful activity for me, but I'm still tied to this person who is making decisions for me and deciding my abilities and deciding and directing my intentionality.
>
> Let's change it a little bit. . . . You don't have to ask my permission and you're going to be going on your own.
>
> But . . . we'll have the annual assessment of your "street crossedness" . . . so if something happens to you when you go across the street to the corner store, it's going to be my fault.

> Well, this is where the rubber meets the road. . . .
> And if . . . an accident occurs where you're struck by
> a vehicle, it's your fault and not mine . . . this is at the
> core of the paradigm shift in service delivery. We're
> going from a system where we consider ourselves still
> responsible for the acts of those we serve, to a system
> where those we serve are responsible for their acts.
>
> And why is this so important? This is important
> because it is at the core of our human dignity. I suggest
> to you that that which makes us most human is our
> ability to enjoy our successes by having the ability to
> own our own failures.[3]

We need to come a long way to embrace such a paradigm shift in
liability concerns with elders. Yet if that terrain can be covered with
the developmentally disabled population, it should be equally possible with our approach to our elders.

For family members, reaching the right balance between risk
and responsibility takes negotiation. It also often requires overcom-
ing great anxiety. One Connecticut agency, the Greater Hartford
Association for Retarded Citizens (HARC), urges families to identify
their worst fears and then test them out against reality. They counsel
them on measured risks and point out that with increased community exposure, even when there is a problem, their clients are usually
met with kindness and compassion. Successes with individuals with
disabilities, just as with elders, comes out of hard work and careful
planning, with risks taken and fears overcome.

Stan Ingersoll, director of HARC resident supports, deepens the
discussion in practical terms, "The dignity of risk is associated with
the dignity of making decisions. . . . If you're going to appreciate
what decision making is about, then you have to live with the good
and the bad. Some of the decisions people make may not work out
well. And that's really difficult. It's difficult for clients and parents,
and for staff members, administrators and the public."[4]

Stan related an episode that illustrates the heart-wrenching nature of decision making and risk taking: "A HARC client had for years wanted to live in Hartford so he'd be closer to his job. He has a physical disability, so he was especially concerned with safety, as were all of us. We helped him evaluate several available apartments, talked to security people, talked to management, and talked with this participant about the pros and cons. HARC would provide drop-in supports. Ultimately the participant decided to move into the apartment he had selected. However, within two weeks, a burglar broke in while he was there and stole his VCR. It was a terrifying experience for him."

Was it a mistake for him to move into the apartment? After the incident, Stan and his staff did a thorough evaluation of the decision making process and concluded it had been handled carefully. The participant had been provided with all the information and direction to make an informed decision. "I think we did a good job, but I feel awful that that happened," said Stan. "It shows how difficult the issues of dignity and risk can be."[5]

In spite of this frightening experience, the participant has made the decision to try again.

He still wants to live in Hartford and with HARC's help is looking for a new and safer apartment. This courageous young man exemplifies the dignity of having personal goals and being willing to overcome obstacles to reach them.

The point of making so much of this discussion of risk is to reduce the likelihood that we as a society have to spend another thirty years retracing steps already traversed in the groundbreaking social movement of deinstitutionalizing those with developmental disabilities. We have now embarked on an elder-citizen movement to provide options to prevent institutionalization for them. It makes no sense to repeat the same mistakes we made with the developmentally disabled. Compared to the developmentally disabled population, this elder cohort, with its acquired limitations, generally is more diverse, more capable, and more accomplished. Yet the obstacles put in the way of letting them live in their own homes or of providing a more independent environment in residential-care facilities are no less formidable. It is critical that we move decisively to rectify this situation. As pointed out elsewhere in this book, our failure to do so will have profound consequences for all sectors of our society.

In the health-care field in which I work, an area of complex medicolegal decision making regarding advanced directives or living wills has been adequately handled by pre-printed forms where an individual can check a box certifying that they "do" or "do not" desire to have CPR performed, a shock delivered to restart his heart, to be placed on a ventilator, or to have intravenous fluids administered. He can also designate someone else to be his decision maker if he is incapacitated.

One's decision to continue to live in one's home is much less complex and more straightforward. One's ability to ask for any service from a home care provider, technology provider, personal care companion, or home repairman should not be more problematic. Arranging these services and making these decisions are often complicated and occasionally mishandled by our elders. But these difficulties should not so often lead to the conclusion to move our elders into institutional care with its drastic consequences. Moreover we should not be confused by liability issues. Some liability burden should fall on the institution, the health care providers, and the family members that take older individuals out of their homes. The team and the approach that tries to assist them to maintain their preexisting living situation should not be held to a higher standard. There are opposing arguments that accompany complex decision making. But attempting to honor the deeply held wishes of one's elders should not carry the majority of the burden of proof and liability.

Clearly with risk comes responsibility. The risks should be measured, the responsibility taken seriously. But to restate Robert Perske, there can be crippling indignity in safety.

And so my message is simply this: Have the courage and the generosity to allow the elders in your life to live their remaining years as independently and freely as possible. Take the time necessary to listen to their concerns. They may scrape their knees, or worse, but they will be living—not just waiting to die.

seventeen

Are We There Yet? Not by a Mile

ONE OF THE MOST FRUSTRATING PARTS of this five-year journey has been trying to explain the slow response to the Maine Approach idea. If someone offered you a solution that provided you much more choice and palatability at a fraction of the cost, why would you not jump at the chance? Having built the better mousetrap, why is the world not beating a path to our door? What is the missing piece of the puzzle?

One reason is that the Maine Approach differs so dramatically from the current models of elder living. It is a departure from the norm that requires us to suspend some long-held beliefs and practices in eldercare, take a few chances, and think and act differently. History shows us, though, that when prevailing systems are stretched to their max, or have become too big and complex to remain true to their original mission, we cling to them all the more. That's the way unhealthy dependencies often work: our problems grow so big that we think only the "tried and true" can help us. But just what is the tried and true of eldercare? It is a system of options based largely on the personal financial profile of the elder. Let's take a look at a few of those profiles.

A very few individuals have the unlimited financial resources to comprehensively retrofit their homes and hire private around-the-clock care and services. They can employ a hard-working, loyal, resourceful team to cook, clean, garden, and help with personal care. Their primary need will be to stay connected to meaningful social interaction and give their lives a continuing sense of purpose. Sometimes their families are diverse enough, attentive enough, and live close enough to meet these other needs; but often they are not.

Many other older individuals and couples have saved enough money through pensions, investments, and home equity to move into retirement communities. These communities offer a spectrum of options, from independent condos, cottages, or apartments to assisted-living facilities and nursing homes on the same premises. Many such complexes offer enticing activities for the more active, and occasionally stretch to meet the changing needs of their residents as they age and need more services. Most, however, conveniently hide many of the important issues of aging that face their members. When that time of needing more services inevitably comes, their members must find other arrangements and move somewhere else. Most such places do not have an approach to continue to engage their members in meaningful living once they become infirm.

Many more individuals have selectively and slowly adjusted their daily patterns to reflect their changing circumstances. They do the best they can to find reliable local individuals to run a few errands, clean the house, do a few household repairs, set their hair, and do their yard work. These individuals prefer their own home to any other living situation. Their financial resources are often quite limited, but they plan and budget carefully and anticipate their future needs. They have the basics covered but give very little thought to the rest of their lives. They are often resigned to the fact that isolation, lone-liness, and lack of ongoing purpose and societal contributions are expected at this stage of their lives.

Most older individuals, though, appear to have no well-defined strategy. They hope to avoid having to face the inevitable. They say they will deal with it when the time comes, and will likely choose not to recognize when that time has actually come. Or they let their children figure things out for them. They defer any decision until there is a crisis. Often their financial resources are very limited: a social security check, perhaps a home fully paid for but in need of repairs and therefore only a small source of equity. These elders rarely think of themselves as having any skills or attributes useful to others. But even this subgroup has many unrecognized abilities that have not been seen outside of the confines of their own home.

For any of these elders or their family members shopping for residential-care services, the sticker shock is numbing. At $50,000 to $100,000 per person per year for assisted-living or nursing home care, most individuals exhaust their personal financial resources in twelve to eighteen months and then rely on state assistance. Many other elders cannot even access any such care from day one without state assistance. The road to this decision point is painful as well.

First of all, savings are often completely depleted. For a generation that saved and sacrificed to navigate the Great Depression, wars, layoffs, economic downturns, raising children and sending them to college, and usually paying bills promptly, this prospect is a bitter reality. If you are part of a couple, often your spouse has different needs and longevity that must be accounted for.

Selling your primary asset, your home of many years, is equally unwelcome, but often the most expedient choice. Depending on your real estate market, and the ever-increasing costs of retirement communities or newer smaller homes, this option is not as attractive as it once was. Executing a reverse mortgage (essentially taking out a home equity loan on the house you worked hard to own debt free) where you spend down the value accumulated over a lifetime is sometimes a bit more palatable. It too faces some of the volatility of the current real estate market when one assesses how much capital can actually be freed up in this way. And as the costs rapidly escalate for the residential care that you can purchase for your spouse or yourself, this solution becomes only a temporary fix.

A serious unintended consequence of these decisions lies in their effect on the financial future of many families. Many elders had visions of leaving money or property to their children or grandchildren. Children have relied on family inheritance for generations. Other seniors wished some of their savings could fund extraordinary expenses for someone in their family: helping a daughter deal with a divorce or an illness, helping a son or grandson finance a car, or supporting a grandchild's aspirations to go to college or start a business. Still others struggle already with taxes, repairs, and medication costs that, altogether, make the golden years a serious financial struggle, not because they were careless with their money, but because they lived too long and had outlived their savings, accumulated at a time when expenses were more manageable. Most people just do not see any alternative to residential care because prior to our Maine Approach, no reasonable option existed.

In addition, we have the relatively recent phenomenon of a "sandwich generation" of adult sons and daughters of aging parents trying to juggle their children's education expenses, their own retirement plans, their own living expenses, and now seeking ways to help support a parent in one of the situations outlined above. It is increasingly difficult to make ends meet financially. The emotional costs of juggling a family, a career, and an aging parent are complicated enough to warrant a book of their own.

And this is one of the kinder scenarios. Often the adult children as "heirs" selfishly quarrel over Mom or Dad spending *their* future inheritance on health care costs, home remodeling, or personal caregivers. Others are in a hurry to move parents into residential care so they can move into or sell their parents' home. Still others begin as well-meaning holders of power-of-attorney letters and after having access to bank accounts and pensions, gradually and often secretly, utilize these funds for their personal financial needs.

Who is there to look out for the elders' best interests? When the deeds are egregious, authorities often get involved but do nothing to restore the lost funds. When it is just poor judgment, everyone looks the other way. Often the misdeeds remain under the radar.

Next to money, the most common issue affecting an elder's options is his or her competence to make his or her own decisions. Who is the ultimate decision maker? Who is in charge? In an ideal world, there would be a measured, gradual transition from generation to generation where the elder shares and eventually turns over responsibility for key household and financial functions to his or her children. Such a transition requires a close working relationship and a minimum of emotional baggage. It requires well-adapted adults and physical proximity to have the opportunity see and know what the elder's wants, needs, and goals might be. We all know most families have significant barriers that preclude any such smooth transition.

For many, insidious memory impairment colludes with preexisting personality traits to produce a messy canvas. By age 85, more than 50 percent of elders have memory issues, and these issues did not start abruptly at age 85.

So when I enter this delicate situation as a concerned adult son or daughter, how is my input going to be received? How do I identify and honor the wishes of my parent(s) if they differ significantly from my own? Likely, their choices will be very different from mine because of the tremendous differences in their lifetime experiences.

Moreover, the spectrum of memory impairment and the decision making that results is broad, and the overlap from one domain of living to another is often illogical, and unpredictable. For a long time, the legal system has dealt with this issue by drafting various documents to delegate authority: power of attorney, medical power of attorney, guardianship, conservators, living-will delegates. None of these instruments help one deal with a parent trying to maintain some control over his or her life. Adult sons and daughters wrestle with understanding their parents' wishes knowing full well that their parents cannot advocate completely for themselves. The current landscape leaves much to be desired.

Here is how the elder is likely to see it: Just because my sense of time is permanently off, so that I do not know what day it is; or just because part of my short-term memory is gone so that I do not remember what I had for breakfast, or whether I had any at all; or just because I continually forget to use my walker or cane, you should not conclude that I do not care about where I live, or that I have no opinion about many other things that are going on around me. I may not be able to spell out for you or with you what I want, but I can surely tell you what I do not want or what I think I do not want. I can certainly weigh in on where I want to live, and how I want to spend the rest of my life. However, my opinion may only be expressed once you have done your best to find some solution for me.

So, again, who is going to act in the elders' best interests?

Kathryn, regardless of her dementia and complete inability to manage her own finances or own care, can gush about Hodgdon Green, "I love it here. We're so lucky to have a place like Hodgdon Green." She wasn't able to find Hodgdon Green on her own, but now that she's there she can express that she's happy. Al, despite no longer driving, and rarely cooking, would live at home on Spam, Fig Newtons, and V8 Juice if someone would provide them. He seems incapable of giving serious thought to the big picture of residential options. He will sidestep the conversation, deny he needs the assistance he requires every day, and insist he is doing fine just as he is. In today's world, many would declare him past the point where he can make rational decisions about his future. "I'd like to stay here and keep doing what I'm doing," is his typical vague response. Yet as unengaged as that may sound, he is actually making a strong statement that he prefers to stay in his own home.

Into this potential hornets' nest step the liability concerns of insurance, financial, and medical institutions. Staying at home in less than ideal circumstances, though desired by 85–95 percent of elders, is not an option that many institutions will condone, let alone bless and assist. Home health agencies see the potential dangers—in other words, liabilities—in the way certain elders are living and step aside. So, hospital-discharge planners, and occupational/physical therapists promote residential care, usually in their own facilities, as being the safest choice. Often their lens is focused on only one aspect of that elder's life, as seen only from the vantage point of someone who may be at least two generations removed from the elder in question.

Caregivers such as doctors and nurses who are very comfortable in such institutional settings do not understand how intimidating, and foreign, residential care is for so many older individuals. They are often intimidating places for people close to an elder, too.

Visitors, whether family or volunteers, immediately sense that they are on someone else's turf, with different, often unstated, rules that often inhibit many necessary interactions. Family members often limit their visits to relatives once they are in a residential-care facility. They do not like to see their loved one in this light but prefer to remember them as he or she used to be. They are often distressed by seeing their loved one with different, more difficult disabilities. It all adds up to quite a scary environment.

As residential caregivers take over more of the activities of daily living, the independence of the residents is dramatically reduced, and an accelerating downward spiral continues. Seeing your loved one decline often creates more emotional distance between the two of you. In the residential-care setting, there may be very little privacy to discuss such difficult topics.

So who is going to advocate for our elders, and how are the issues of financial and legal responsibility to be negotiated? With all the roadblocks noted above, many family members give up on trying to find innovative ways to help their aging loved ones carry on fulfilling lives. It becomes far easier and less guilt producing to simply follow the tide of institutional advice. Yet people rarely understand that advice is driven more by concerns about finances and liability than quality of life.

Caregivers, though, have the opportunity to change this dynamic. Until we can honestly say that residential care is so appealing that we would willingly change places with those elders residing there, we medical personnel must be more willing to entertain, promote, and develop more comprehensive stay-at-home options for our elders. We also must try much harder to make residential care reflect a much richer daily life than just a version of a hospital stay.

The paradigm presented by the Maine Approach goes a very long way toward addressing these challenges. But, without the backing of more caregivers who see their value, we can't expect elders and their families to know of these options, or experiment with them.

So why aren't more hospital case workers and family physicians and social service agencies suggesting alternatives like the Maine Approach to the families who are depending on their every word of advice? Given the financial challenges faced by state and federal governments in meeting imminent projected residential-care needs, interest in an alternative approach should be high. Change is always difficult, but there is an additional challenge: many think such an approach is just unrealistic. They don't see a way around the current institutional norms and existing governmental regulations. They want to see the Maine Approach stand the test of time under additional scrutiny. But I believe most individuals in these organizations also aspire to a better paradigm. They just do not know how to get there.

Caregivers also need to get serious about the fact that the current residential-care system is doomed to failure. A bad business model does not get better just because you do it faster or in greater volume.

I have given no fewer than a hundred presentations over the last five years to medical staffs, hospital CEOs and senior management teams, hospital reorganization retreats, home-health agency seminars, discharge planners, retirement community managers, administrators of nursing homes and assisted-living facilities, senior service organizations, local branches of national service organizations, foundation funders, human-services agency commissioners, directors of elder service bureaus, legislators and other elected officials and their staff, leaders at geriatric education centers at colleges and medical schools, local business groups, and local women's groups. The reception everywhere has been universally welcoming. The response to most of the new paradigm and its components has been one of general encouragement.

To cope humanely with the coming age wave, it seems clear to me that we need to put many more affordable choices within the reach of a much greater portion of the elder population. So, in these talks I have shown how the ElderCare Network developed an approach that costs up to *90 percent* less than the current alternatives. For those who cannot afford even this greatly reduced expenditure, the governments and benevolent organizations that are called on to assist with payment can see their financial resources dramatically extended when the vast majority of elder individuals can stay in their own homes or move into the noninstitutional surroundings of their neighbors' homes. Imagine, I ask them, what could happen if long-term-care insurance policies started to recognize alternative at-home options.

But, ironically, the idea of saving someone money is not very well received—even saving their own institutional money.

For example, several state agencies feared that incorporating our ideas and dramatically reducing the cost of their client care would reduce the state or federal dollars coming to their organization. They would rather continue to provide a more expensive, inferior service than see their funding potentially reduced. Others were concerned that blazing a new trail would require too much reform of the regulatory and payment systems that governed their world. They were not interested in incurring the expense of proposing new approaches. Most organizations wanted only to see a new revenue stream immediately without any attendant development costs or other investment on their part.

Doing more with less just did not compute. Since many of these organizations are in the public sector, taking risks or investing in new products or innovation are not in the skill sets they have developed over the years.

Many others were simply unconcerned about impending crises that they hoped would arrive after they had moved on to their next job or retired. Many must answer to boards whose directors were risk averse especially when proposing a model not yet replicated. So despite their apparent genuine interest in our model, they were uniformly too busy with other parts of their jobs to embrace something this new and this complex.

Several others have suggested that a big reason for delays in accepting our approach is others' own self-interest or greed. Many suspect that the approach I have outlined threatens the residential-care industrial complex.

Of course the opposite is true. With several of the components and processes employed in our packages, assisted-living facilities will be able to reduce their costs, enhance their appeal to customers, and retain their residents longer by stretching their personnel resources. Nursing facilities can similarly reduce their costs, and enrich their programs without incurring new expense. Their bottom lines will improve. Given the gray tsunami soon upon us, there will be plenty of business for every enterprise willing to focus energy and investment on this elderly cohort. However, the Maine Approach will reduce the need to build five to ten times as many residential-care facilities. Realistically, we may only need twice as many as we currently have.

Still others point to the inherent divide between the nonprofit and for-profit institutions that currently provide eldercare. They both compete with, and complement, one another. They have similar missions in the public eye, but different economic motives. Even so, improving efficiency, elder satisfaction, and delivering more services for less should matter equally to both sectors. As one astute nonprofit executive told me, "If you're going to succeed anywhere—nonprofit or for-profit—you're going to have to have a well-oiled machine."

Some conversations about roadblocks even reflect the general skepticism of our age. An economic aide to a senior U.S. senator warned me that the Maine Approach was too democratic, too liberal, and that it would not play well in the current political climate. Senior members of a financial investment house warned that as soon as I was successful enough or the approach visible enough, I would be bought out. This, they explained, meant the Maine Approach could spread, and current more profitable ways of serving this market could be threatened. It seems ironic that some of the kings of capitalism would have so little faith in the business power of a new idea.

This kind of cynicism is neither helpful nor appropriate. There are many examples of successful socially responsible businesses. Likewise, there are innumerable examples coming out of corporate boardrooms illustrating how serving the community better

improves the company's bottom line. We are in the midst of rework-
ing the conventional wisdom of what works in American business. A
growing number of books examine the potential metamorphosis of
corporations into profit-making drivers of much-needed progress—
on environmental, social, and cultural fronts. In fact, today's leading
thinkers on socially responsible business models argue that doing it
any differently will lead to failure of one's business.

That brings me to the final obstacle. What we propose when we
discuss the Maine Approach defies the assembly-line thinking that
has driven health care for the past fifty years. It is messy, a little
chaotic, and demands that we be able to adjust frequently to the
changing requirements and even whims of our clients. It cannot be
otherwise, because we are attempting to address the needs of the
majority of older individuals, regardless of income, interest, or ability. It is a quilt, not a silk sheet. Each component of the program can
be utilized and shaped in many different ways. But although it has
many parts, none of them are inherently complicated. Our approach
involves assembling these many simple pieces into an effective,
whole package. It demands hands-on observation and customiza-
tion. But that doesn't mean it can't be spread far and wide.

Indeed, even as we listen to fears about change, or competition with
existing infrastructure, we often hear from progressive, far-thinking
agencies and nonprofits that understand the Maine Approach could
help their communities dramatically reduce their need to build large
numbers of new residential-care facilities and retirement communities. They understand that relatively few dollars could be expended
to upgrade existing private residences rather than build larger, more
impersonal facilities. And, most of all, they understand that this
approach not only preserves the independence of many elders for a
longer period of time, but also gives many elders a renewed sense of
purpose.

To bring our model to these and other communities in and outside
of Maine, we have formed a limited-profit enterprise called Full
Circle America. Our goal is to create turnkey operations modeled

on the Maine Approach that can be implemented readily and reliably by our affiliates anywhere the need exists. As these early adopters add their own features to the program, improvements will continue. No doubt the technology tools that we have employed over the last few years will continue to be improved and will become even less expensive.

Already, in early 2011, we have signed on a few other communities in Maine and plans are under way for other East Coast communities. As soon as a dozen or so affiliates are up and running, we will be on our way.

And so we carry on despite the reluctance of so many to change course when it is so much easier to follow the others over the cliff. The goal remains, though, to herd the cliff walkers away from the edge. We've all heard, "If you build it they will come." Slowly but steadily, they *are* coming. There is simply no better way to meet the challenge.

eighteen

Alone and Invisible Too: The Next Generation

FOR THE NEAR TERM, THE ADULT SONS and daughters of aging parents hold an important key that will determine whether any new model of eldercare is embraced widely in the United States. Having been raised in a more permissive and self-indulgent era than their parents, many adult children possess the proper empathy for their aging parents but have been reluctant to assume a responsive and responsible role in their decision-making process. Like many struggling with other common social problems, they often see the issue only as their own personal problem. Adult children, therefore, are also isolated, alone, and invisible as they confront their parents' situation.

There are many factors that contribute to this current state of poor family communication. Let's start with the aging parents. Having been raised in the shadow of the Great Depression, they have low expectations for any extras in their lives. Having been taught to be self-reliant, they are loath to ask for or accept any help. They were often imbued with a mind-set of sacrificing their lives for the next generation. After a lifetime of giving all of their resources to make their children's success possible, they cannot conceive of asking their children to support them financially. They refuse to complicate their children's lives by asking them to deal with their declining years. While these same elders may have seen their own parents' generation willingly accept taking an aging family member or in-law into their own homes for the rest of their lives, such a course is anathema to them. "They have their own lives," my older patients regularly remark when talking about their children. In many instances, they have seen firsthand the profound alteration of family life that ensued. They do not wish to replicate that chain of events. Throughout their careers, they have often planned for their future, lived with greater financial opportunity than previous generations, and never expected to outlive their savings. They also never expected to have to rely on their own children later in life.

Yet they have not noticed that family options can now be quite different. Our homes and our communities have the potential to more easily accommodate a variety of scenarios. The technology, conveniences, and services of the twenty-first century make it possible to envision and then implement a solution that does not need to replicate the difficulties that the older generation fears.

From the point of view of the adults in the sandwich generation, the elder landscape is hazy. The path is not yet blazed. Solutions require problem solving and social engineering in a major way. Elder services require commitment of time and financial resources at a time when both are already in short supply. Frankly, many adult children are too busy, too greedy, or too oblivious to attend to what is going on. Others are far too easily falsely reassured by their frail, failing parents that everything is okay.

Bill and Anita live far off the beaten path in a picturesque log home they built on a lake when Bill first retired with a reasonable corporate pension. All five children live out of state, and through a variety of complicated family dynamics, their contact is now very limited. What Bill and Anita consider a close relationship is a phone call from one of the children every month, and a summer visit from another every year. As self-sufficient and admirably stalwart as Bill and Anita try to be, they could sorely benefit from a much more involved family or significant others as they struggle to make some very complicated decisions.

Bud was a successful cartoonist who kept working until he was 85. After his wife died, his dog, his work, and cocktail hour were his main interests. He enjoyed his neighbors' occasional visits, and met a few new people. But his mother's early rejection of his talents, and the lack of role models in his vaudeville days made him a bit of a loner. He was proud of his son but knew no way to show it. He did not want to bother him with his life or his concerns. He'd solve his problems on his own.

Many parent–adult child relationships remain almost irreparably strained from earlier family conflict. If that parent was too stern a disciplinarian, vehemently disapproved of a marriage or a divorce, disagreed about moves, job choices, or child-rearing approaches, relationships became strained, ties severed, or broad gulfs formed. The wounds may not have healed, and that kindly, engaging 90-year-old before us is not the individual that those out-of-state children remember. Many members of that generation gave you what they thought you needed to launch you and then let go. They did not know "that nurturing thing" that is now a customary part of child rearing and that now promotes "keeping in touch" with adult children once they leave the nest.

Kim's dad drove a truck and Jill's worked for the railroad. They were absent from the home and from their children's lives for extended periods of time. Now as they contemplate helping their older fathers cope with major decisions, they realize they don't know them very well. The same holds true for children separated from one parent or the other by divorce. The emotional bonds that many families take for granted are by no means universal.

We can't expect a dysfunctional family all of a sudden to come together, heal their old wounds, be gracious and caring, and work together to solve issues in uncharted territory. This is a very tall order that demands that there be other advocates for elders in the discussion.

As Francine Russo pointed out in *Time* magazine, caring for an aging parent can reignite sibling tensions. "When my mother's health was failing, I was the 'bad' sister who lived far away and wasn't involved," wrote Russo.

I was widowed, raising kids and working, but that wasn't really why I kept to weekly calls and short, infrequent visits. I was stuck in my adolescent role as the aloof achiever, defending myself from my judgmental mother and other family craziness. As always, I deflected my sister's digs about not being around more—and I didn't hear her rising desperation. . . .

"It's like being put down with your siblings in the center of a nuclear reactor and being told, 'Figure it out,'" says University of Colorado geropsychologist Sara Honn Qualls.

Eldercare and end-of-life debates often hit families after decades of negotiating nothing more serious than where to spend Thanksgiving. We can be grown-ups with successful careers and kids of our own, yet all the old stuff ambushes us: sibling rivalry, entrenched roles and resentments, the way our family talked or didn't talk about important things.[1]

Still others are deeply committed to a parent's welfare and are exhausted trying to help. One of the most poignant portrayals of this side of the coin is the article by Jonathan Rausch in the *Atlantic* entitled "Letting Go of My Father." Rausch's 80-year-old father insisted he could live independently on the other side of the country. A proud man, a retired, highly respected lawyer, he struggled mightily with the activities of daily living due to his medical problems stemming from an aggressive form of Parkinson's disease. But he refused help. Eventually Rausch moved his father to an apartment near him on the East Coast. His father's multiple-system atrophy progressed rapidly and motor control worsened. He writes, "I came to dread the ring of the telephone: it might be my father on the floor, asking me to come over and pick him up, or it might be emergency medical services, summoned by a neighbor or the call button. Once, when I arrived amid a commotion of paramedics and flashing lights, a neighbor, her face flushed with fear, yelling to me, 'He can't live here! You've got to move him!' In the midst of it all, my father would be entreating everyone to leave him be. My professional work all but stopped."

Finally, when his partner tried to take his dad shopping, and his dad became stiff and incoherent in the grocery aisle and then didn't remember anything about the incident, Jonathan snapped, "That was the day I realized that he could not cope and I could not cope and, emotionally, he could take me down with him. And I discovered in myself an awful determination not to let that happen." It was at that point that Rausch entered the difficult terrain that many children find themselves in: of trying to make a parent do something the parent adamantly opposes—such as moving into a facility—in order to preserve his own sanity, or lifestyle, or even his livelihood.

He then eloquently catalogs his discovery of all the practical wisdom he collected on the street from coworkers, acquaintances, and other professionals. Finally, Rausch appealed to his father as a father—admitting that being his de facto caretaker was simply too much for him, and his father, being a good father, agreed to make the move that would make his son's life more manageable.

"How can it be that so many people like me are so completely unprepared for what is, after all, one of life's near certainties?" asked Rausch. "I am now convinced that millions of middle-aged Americans need more help than they are getting, and that the critical step toward solving the problem is a cultural change akin to the one demanded by the feminists in the 1960s. . . . [T]oday's invisible caregivers . . . are being asked to do alone and out of sight what in fact requires not just private sympathy and toleration but public acknowledgment and proactive assistance."[2]

Amen. There are so many important feelings and themes presented in that article. I encourage everyone to read it. Rausch accurately depicts how all-absorbing it can be to manage a significant portion of an aging parent's life. Then the lack of cooperation, lack of appreciation, and lack of support in the rest of one's life pushes the caregiving adult child to the brink of despair.

There are other important issues that stand in the way of adult children being a better advocate for a parent. Money heads that list. Anthony and Ellen, like so many other older couples, incorrectly assume that Medicare or Medicaid or some other state or federal agency will pay for the services that they need. They do not understand that eldercare is so costly that no one wants to tackle it. They do not grasp that state assistance only comes into play after all one's private funds have been spent and they are destitute. And even then, though they may be eligible for services or even residential care, finding people or facilities to provide such care at the paltry reimbursements offered by Medicaid is difficult, and waiting lists grow longer.

Some adult children encourage their parents to spend their savings and their home equity to provide the things they need and want later in life. Others have arranged to have the financial assets of the parents turned over to them, and are quick to plan to have the aging parent placed in a state-supported facility even against the parent's stated wishes. Our society must encourage the creation of other recognized advocates for many elders. Whether this function is performed by community-based church leaders or social workers functioning as mediators, there should be a venue within the community for such difficult dynamics to be hammered out. Expecting dysfunctional families to come together to serve the elders' best interests is unrealistic.

Other workable advocates may occasionally appear. In my own community, Charlie started out as an energetic retiree helping a neighbor, 88-year-old Dorothy, with some projects around her home. She had lost one son to cancer and burned the bridge to the other child. Charlie grew very fond of her. Little by little, as Dorothy's health worsened, it became apparent that Charlie's special combination of coaxing, complementing, and teasing produced results that no other caregiver could duplicate. He and his wife now devote a major part of their lives to caring for Dorothy. They have overcome many legal and familial obstacles to see that Dorothy's needs are

well met. They bring a renewed richness into her life, and she recip-
rocates with her appreciation. It is not always formal training that
is necessary. Such care requires commitment and heart. Sometimes
that can emanate more easily from those without blood relationship
to a particular elder.

Many elders in various communities across the United States are
turning to each other for support, jointly contracting for services,
and creating new support systems. Beacon Hill Village in Boston
and its imitators are virtual communities that are connecting neighbors in various ways for group benefit. Some friends are even step-
ping up to challenge decisions made by well-meaning adult children
to move their friends out of their own homes and into residential
care. At times it takes such advocacy to stop a sequence of events
unpalatable to an aging parent because that parent is reluctant to
express her true feelings to her own children.

Where can we look for guidance to navigate this apparently
uncharted territory? In 1997, Edwin J. Pittock founded an organization called the Society of Certified Senior Advisors to promote
in-depth, standardized education for ethical, honest, and princi-
pled professionals who work with seniors. They have developed a
dynamic organization with a comprehensive course curriculum.
Their mission is to train professionals from all walks of life to understand the special needs of aging individuals and commit to serving
them well in their particular line of work.

Other organizations like the Family Caregiver Alliance (www
.caregiver.org); The National Alliance for Caregiving (www.care
giving.org); and a bulletin board sponsored by Johnson and Johnson
(strengthforcaring.com) provide other starting points. And, of
course, the Full Circle America (www.FullCircleAmerica.com) solution, which we hope to replicate in 10,000 American communities
over the next decade, is driven by the notion that each community
possesses an army of potential partners to address the wide array
of needs and aspirations of an aging population. This approach is
heavily dependent upon the participation of family and volunteers to

share the load and in doing so help to relieve the financial and time commitment required of any one family member or volunteer.

In the process we can all rediscover the joys of multigenerational connections—whether with our own parents, or with other elders. In fact, it may be through the eyes, and hearts, and minds of other elders that we come to know our own parents better. As a community, we can find the support that we desire to meet our own needs. In the process, we just might learn that the solutions for our elders also provide a cure for our own loneliness and invisibility.

nineteen

Rolling It Out Nationally, Reaping Additional Rewards

IF YOU HAVE MADE IT THIS FAR, I hope it is a sign that you are interested in helping solve the eldercare crisis. And we will need your help.

The numbers are daunting. Assume for a moment Full Circle America (FCA) could establish a new, 100-member local Maine Approach affiliate every day of the year for ten years. At the end of that decade we would have 3,650 locations serving 365,000 elders. Nice. But that would barely scratch the surface when closer to 10 million elders will need care across the nation by the end of that decade. If we are more ambitious, and set the bar at 1,000 local offices per year for ten years, we will be serving 1 million elders. Better. And with luck and persistence, by the year 2030 we may be able to reach every elder in the country.

So our ambitious, albeit still inadequate, goal is to roll out the Maine Approach to 10,000 communities over the next ten years, with the services delivered through independently owned and operated local affiliates. We believe we can help any diligent adult, at any age, to launch an affiliate. For those who pass the screening and training (which we will pay for), we will provide all of the administrative support and even seed capital to help get the local affiliate off the ground and serving others. Significant barriers to adoption and rapid growth must be eliminated if our country is going to avert the social and economic disaster caused by ignoring the approaching gray tsunami. In addition to providing help for those first million elders, the FCA program will create a significant small-business opportunity for those seeking to open and manage a local affiliate.

An essential part of executing the Maine Approach vision is to find a reasonable way to distribute the model. From the beginning, it has been apparent that the success of a new approach to eldercare will require the endorsement of an elder's trusted advisors. Making such big decisions about where to live and how to live is much more intimate than buying a product or a service. It requires education and encouragement to face your future in your declining years with an optimism that you have choice, options, good years ahead, something to offer, purpose and value to impart. To convey such sentiments and stimulate active decision making will take skilled professionals who can also embrace flexibility and choice.

Those of us in health care who know and love elders, and want to advocate for them, have hoped to get them to make changes proactively. We have sought a way to avert the last-minute-crisis decision making that is so much a part of the landscape today. But up until now there have not been many good options to promote.

Small primary-care offices seem a natural source of community leadership. The medical community is now abuzz with its latest catchphrase, the "medical home." Essentially, the policy makers are saying that in this era of super-subspecialization and six-minute doctor's visits, patients need someone in the health-care world to coordinate their care, and give advice. Navigating such complexity in a holistic way is very important and should be paid for. The last part, the payment system, is the sticking point because the system is already broken and no one wants to give up their nickel to make this desirable piece happen.

Despite the financial challenges, family physicians in many communities have been playing this role since the field became a specialty in the 1960s. Many are looking for better ways to enhance their ability to meet their patients' needs in this institutionalized and increasingly impersonal world we call health care. I was one of them.

In 2003, when three family physicians and I founded our private practice, Full Circle Family Medicine, we took the bold step to leave a large, institutional multispecialty practice because too much of our energies were consumed by meetings with middle management about the business of medicine rather than patient care. We also believed that it is our ethical responsibility to serve the whole community irrespective of a patient's ability to pay.

Today our seven providers and eight support staff deliver high-quality, much-sought-after care to 6,000 Lincoln County residents, of whom 18 percent are MaineCare (Medicaid) recipients, close to 25 percent are on Medicare, 10 percent are self-pay (or delayed pay) uninsured, and the remaining third have commercial insurance. About 1,500 of our patients are seniors. Daily we wrestle with the challenges of many proud, but increasingly frail elders wanting to stay in their own homes, yet who are isolated from dispersed and busy families and lonely from losses of spouses and friends.

However, they crave more human contact and the opportunity to still be a useful member of the community. Additionally, each year we are more constrained by a broken, corporate, health-care system that increasingly produces a flat revenue stream and, most importantly, restricts our ability to provide holistic, personalized care that could address their needs.

Family physicians are ideally suited by their training and experience to help promote the Maine Approach in their communities. With 94,000 members of the American Academy of Family Physicians, we indeed have the workforce to address these burgeoning elder needs. With the proven adaptability of our profession over the last twenty years, I have no doubt that we can incorporate these elements into many office practices without much work, especially if a turnkey model and full support services are provided by FCA.

So, in our search for 10,000 community leaders that can roll out the Maine Approach, family physicians rank high among the potential community members that can spearhead an affiliate. They have earned the trust of their elder patients. They have the stature in their communities. Many have the small-business and innovation skills to enhance the basic Maine Approach and fine-tune it to suit the local culture and language. However, others connected to the current fabric of eldercare in their communities are also in a good position to connect with local services and local caregivers and get a network off the ground. Anyone so motivated can find more information about Full Circle America and our affiliate program in the appendix of this book. That information is further elaborated on our website, where you can find everything from organizational protocols to job descriptions to descriptions of available packages for eldercare.

My hope is that by spreading the Maine Approach, we will not only transform the way our society interacts with its elders, we also—as preposterous as it may sound—help save America. How so?

First, we correct our downward spiral in eldercare and arrest the mounting costs of continuing with such a broken system. Each small county or community of 50,000 people faces the near-term prospect of spending $100 million to build and $50 million per year to maintain additional residential-care facilities that most people dread. So any approach that holds the promise of a different outcome should be seriously examined. The profound and widespread ramifications of a new eldercare paradigm can contribute to a rebirth of many other sectors of our country, which is truly exciting. The opportunity goes way beyond its narrow and most obvious benefits.

Since the percentage of the U.S. population over 65 years old is rapidly approaching 25 percent of the total population, any fundamental change directly affects one in four people. You do not need to do much extrapolation to see that each one of these seniors has an effect on his or her children and grandchildren, on neighbors, on those workers that provide services to them, on those that interact with them at the church, the store, the theater, the restaurant. In effect, the whole community is not very far removed from their entire local senior cohort.

By empowering this disenfranchised, warehoused, and abandoned group to retake control of their lives and to begin again to contribute to the rich fabric of their community, the Maine

Approach can have a deeply transformational impact on the rest of our society as well.

If we could apply just some of the Maine Approach to the medical system, for instance, we could help it become more holistic, more transparent, and more affordable—goals our society has had for decades. Patients have long wanted to participate more fully in their own health care, and physicians and policy makers seek ways to make patients take more personal responsibility for their own health. The path to a more individualized, always modifiable, easily accessible, and far more affordable model runs straight through the same paradigm we've laid out for eldercare reform. The possibility of harnessing the Internet, video calling, and videoconferencing to serve so many unique individuals in each community greatly expands the concepts already touched on by WebMD, online health chat rooms, and telemedicine applications.

A move toward more community-based care could also reenergize primary care medicine, and attract more people to all aspects of it. For a long time, the health-care industry's technology, innovation, research, and money has all been focused on the subspecialties of the medical-care world. It is time for that lopsided approach to change and time for those resources to flow into primary care.

Moreover, variations on the Maine model can be applied to address the needs of other marginalized subgroups, as well—such as the intellectually challenged. Addressing the needs of this large cohort is certainly no more complicated than addressing those of our elders, though the regulatory mess to be untangled is likely harder. Many of the individuals who work in this field come out of a professional training model that has promoted deinstitutionalization their entire careers. I think they can be a wonderful resource to promote the principles and implementation of something similar to the Maine Approach for their clients and organizations. They also have a deep interest in seeing that a different approach is available for their aging clients, as these individuals do not fit easily into traditional elder residential care.

The departments of disability and vocational rehabilitation also have much to gain from our work. Many counselors in this field report that the ideal job-retraining opportunity that they seek for many of their clients is a computer-based job that the client can perform from home without the attendant transportation issues. The eldercare paradigm we envision has many opportunities for those with physical disabilities to have meaningful and gainful employment. In fact, as I write this, our most experienced and dedicated tele-caregiver is a physically disabled man supervising many elders from his home. He is very grateful to be contributing again to his community.

My hope is that if we can expand our small grassroots effort widely enough to address our national eldercare crisis, that success could help us see that other intractable problems may also not be so impossible to address after all. Our country needs to rediscover its former "can-do" attitude if it is going to continue to prosper. Part of developing that attitude will lie in our ability to harness the innate talent and experience of all of our community members, and create new coalitions that work cooperatively on other local issues.

Let's consider how an empowered group of elders might come together to reengage in their communities and tackle some serious problems brewing there. Many forecasters look at the need for significant educational reform to provide the foundation for any national economic rebirth. The Maine Approach, expanded nationally, holds enormous potential to intersect with these educational-system needs in many ways. Elders are an untapped hidden resource for schools in need. They can help students in elementary school develop reading and spelling skills—either in the classroom itself or via remote video technology that can easily bring their resources into the school or home. When middle-school or junior-high students need mentors, or remedial tutors, many elders can similarly offer their talents, again remotely if necessary. When high school students need their intergenerational connections with elders to provide insight into the social studies, history, or literature worlds that the elders may have personally witnessed, the elders stand ready to participate. When the troubled student at any age needs a cool head, or perhaps just a concerned outsider with some time and some interest to help him or her get through a messy stage of development, or when such a youth lacks the relationships at home to relate to him or her at that time, again our elder cohort can play a role. Web-based learning at sites like Tutorvista, or mentoring sites available online, are already providing such services to a select group of users. There is no reason this approach cannot be greatly expanded.

The costs to develop such a distributed model of reform are comparatively cheap and can be incorporated into the technological spine of the elder-at-home model. Such a technology-based enhancement can be used as a springboard for a broader effort of community educating community. Many other older adults, after a productive career in their chosen field, are ready to give back in the second half of their lives in a meaningful way. They can be similarly enlisted to work either with elders or with other youth or young adults through such a technology platform. Groups like Big Brothers/Big Sisters, the Foster Grandparent Program, and Service Corps of Retired Executives (SCORE) can extend their good work by being connected to an elder social network.

Local governments are also missing out on the potential contributions of their community elders. With broadband availability and public-access TV, there is no reason that our community elders cannot continue to participate in their town meetings, as well as select-board and planning-board meetings. Many had lifelong roles in public service but no longer can attend meetings. Many have a broad range of experience to bring to bear on specific issues. At a time when many small towns have poor turnout at such meetings and solutions chosen seem often to lack our collective wisdom, such an approach could reinvigorate the process, and encourage broader participation. Many other local organizations, from town libraries, arts councils, and service organizations, would also benefit from making it easier for their community's elders to participate.

FCA has also had some enthusiastic responses from U.S. veterans' groups seeking ways to have younger servicemen connect with their older veterans for mutual benefit. These veterans' groups also want a different future for those older veterans in their care; they are not content with the eldercare choices available at Veterans' Homes and Hospitals.

Perhaps the biggest impact of changing the paradigm in elder-care will be in that of job creation. As the United States struggles with unusually high unemployment, and few employers are willing to gamble on what industries will have new orders what quarter, eldercare services offer a growth industry destined to be robust for twenty-five to forty years. The needs will be in diverse areas that are accessible to most communities right now with the skill sets and educational levels that already exist in abundance.

A very large support economy will develop around the basic at-home needs of a rapidly enlarging elder cohort. According to current esti-mates, the elder residential-care market will be 20 million caregivers shy of the number needed by 2030. To address this shortfall, we need to create a "guardian angel" workforce—individuals who are a combi-nation of surrogate son or daughter, neighbor, confidant, advocate, life coach, and problem solver. While schooled in the basics of PSS and CNA courses by retired nurses, they will have an expanded focus on utilizing remote monitoring via webcams and motion sensors to promote efficiency and transparency and reduce cost, as well as elder advocacy to empower elders to remain independent and connected to family and community interests. They will not fill the narrow role of a home health agency aide. They will promote true "quality of life" for elder customers by seeking out and fulfilling the needs and wants of that elder in a very broad sense. We estimate a ratio of one "guard-ian angel" per fifty elder members. They will be the cornerstones of the success of our approach. They embody the reason many choose to work in such health-care-related fields: to serve others.

There will be plenty of other jobs to go around, as well. As a matter of fact, we will need to work much smarter just to meet the projected demand. Many of the service-sector jobs will be in personal care, light to heavy supervision, meal preparation, housekeeping, home repair, lawn care, transportation, and basic bookkeeping. Newer services will be in equipment setup and maintenance, mental gymnastics and exercise fitness, and physical therapy aides. With appropriate screening and attention to detail, combined with task-oriented and customer-specific scheduling, elder needs can be met in a satisfying and affordable fashion not now readily available. Many potential employees seeking flexible jobs, including other elders, stay-at-home moms, and those seeking part-time work, can be accommodated in the network envisioned.

For many more elders to stay at home, a lot of house retrofitting will be required. The entire gamut of the building trades will be required including carpenters, plumbers, and electricians. The housing stock already exists, but few planned ahead to live on one floor or to find new ways to navigate between levels. These are jobs that cannot be outsourced overseas.

The model will require building a better community information-technology infrastructure. Hardware, software, and data transfer options will need to continue to evolve. Troubleshooters to problem solve at homes and throughout the network will be essential. Ramping up video technology, creating smart computer learning modules, bringing new video applications to bear on integrating a whole community will be critical to the success of the model. Opportunities for those with technology-based skills will be limitless. VPN hosts will help elders navigate their remote worlds. This entire movement will push the current IT world beyond just additional personal consumption, marketing, and convenience services. Those services that enhance individuals' abilities to share, connect, and help meet more personal and profound human needs will be promoted.

Transportation is the greatest need of robust "stay at home" support services. Current community resources are primarily spent transporting individuals to medical appointments, leaving no services outside of urban areas to allow someone to remain active in community and service organizations, let alone attend arts offerings or sports events. Group trips to flower shows, foliage tours, Christmas shopping, and concerts are always well attended but very rarely offered. We will need a combination of bus routes, shuttles, taxi services, group charters, and a robust volunteer network of drivers to offer elders a full menu of services for all income levels.

As more people age in place, they will need more help with simple tasks from picking up the mail or newspaper to grocery shopping and ordering and getting medication refills. They'll need help with laundry, or replacement parts or even takeout food. At FCA, we focus on meeting these needs with a combination of volunteers and staff working at hours that allow them to continue their schooling, raise families, or have supplemental income.

In many of these cases, elders themselves can fill these new job roles. This is particularly true for errand and handyman services. I often hear from my patients that they have had to neglect simple repairs because reliable workers for small projects are hard to come by. Most contractors do not want these jobs. Yet many older workers and retirees of all ages have a lifetime of skills to offer their peers. And most want to find ways to spend their time meaningfully. For instance, in Maine we've planned a community painting crew to rejuvenate public and other essential community properties like schools, churches, and libraries—and an energy retrofitting crew to weatherproof homes. Elder volunteers can also create cemetery maintenance crews to provide a service many towns lack. All of these efforts would be self-sustaining or income producing once set up.

But perhaps one of the most innovative new roles for elders will be in providing a home away from home for their peers. As you read in earlier chapters, there are many reasons why an elder might need temporary room and board. Their heat may have turned off; their spouses might be are ill or away; or their primary caregiving family member has another commitment due to work, hobbies, children, or vacation. Full Circle America affiliates can link together a network of spare bedrooms from elder homeowners utilizing digital technologies and support services to convert underutilized capacity into a new revenue stream for elder homeowners and an additional care option for the community. The revenue generated allows homeowners to supplement fixed incomes or pay taxes or undertake overdue repairs that will allow them to stay in their own homes longer. It can also provide new meaning and new friendships. We expect this program to be one of the largest revenue producers for affiliates to use to reinvest in the community.

There's also tremendous opportunity in expanding the catering services available to elders—providing a healthy, diverse menu and improving socialization. Again, elders themselves have much to share here. Today's elders possess a variety of food-growing, cooking, and preserving skills that are becoming less common in our communities. There are also many peers that lack the skills to manage capably in the kitchen. Selected elders and older workers can mentor other elders as they adjust to living alone or with diabetes and heart disease, or adjust to arthritis. Others can mentor a younger generation. The fruits of these labors can be made available to elders as an adjunct to Meals on Wheels, as well as increasing the visibility of their talents as they provide product to churches and civic organizations for their meetings.

The possibilities are endless. Elders could help community service organizations and nonprofits get the manpower they need to run their events. They can help pass along traditional crafts—like sewing, quilting, embroidery, and knitting. And, they can help young mothers who often need capable help for a few hours a few times a week while they attend to other duties at home or run errands. Many daycare centers have already pioneered in the use of elder volunteers to supplement their skilled staff. Many elders in the residential-care settings rarely see a baby and become very capable assistants when given the opportunity. With another age group, after-school sitters are often needed by working two-parent families and single working moms to minimize the time their latchkey kids are unsupervised after school. These needs mesh again with the desires of many seniors who live at such a distance from extended families that they rarely see elementary and high school students. Our local experiment has already initiated lunch programs at the elementary and high school where elders are hosted by specific school groups. These events have led to continuing friendships that could be the basis for further collaboration.

All of this, though, is just a superficial look at the transformational domino effect of addressing eldercare according to a new paradigm. In reality, this effort could produce enormous savings over business as usual—all while creating new jobs, new volunteer opportunities, new community collaborations, and new economic value. At a time when political discussion is heavily focused on health-care costs, job creation, and our national debt, it is instructive to return to the starkly different choices we face.

Business as usual, that is using residential care facilities such as nursing homes and assisted living homes as the primary option for eldercare, at our current national utilization rate, will require that most communities construct at least three times as many nursing home beds and eight times as many assisted living beds over the next twenty years. The aggregate cost to build these facilities at today's prices is $1 trillion. The annual operating costs for these facilities will be about $500 billion ($0.5 trillion). As a means of comparison, the total current United States spending on health care from all sources is about $2.5 trillion. And the money spent in this scenario only serves five percent of the over-65 population, and provides a choice most do not want.

The Maine Approach creates a very different economic outcome. It uses a blend of volunteer and paid service providers as well as a unique focus on task management that mixes many part-time contributions and produces the equivalent of one local full-time job for every ten seniors served in the network. These jobs are likely to be in the fields outlined above. Let's extrapolate those numbers on a national scale. For a projected U.S. senior population of 85 million by the year 2030, this approach could yield 8.5 million new jobs—a number equal to the number of American jobs lost since our current economic recession hit in 2007. If we can do this work even more efficiently and serve 25 seniors with one new full-time job, the total of new jobs created nationally still approaches 3.5 million.

In my own Lincoln County in Maine, a county of 35,000 people, this approach can create an additional $6 million of new economic value. If we replicated this phenomenon in every other U.S. community of 35,000 people, it would produce the staggering sum of $60 billion annually of new economic value across the nation. This growth would generate stable well-paying local jobs with benefits and small business money stimulating the local economy of each community. The value of the volunteer component of the Maine approach is also mind-boggling. If 10 percent of those individuals over 65 contribute four hours per week to a meaningful activity, the dollar value for such efforts nationally is about $50 billion annually. If 25 percent participate, the value exceeds $125 billion per year. As mentioned earlier, the full-time job equivalents of this labor pool rival the largest employer in nearly every community and would well exceed a million full-time job equivalents nationally. These calculations should again put in perspective how enormous the demographic and economic implications are of how we as a society choose to advance the cause of eldercare in this country.

The grassroots movement that could make such a turnaround possible can grow, but it will take the hard work of pioneering caregivers and others to get it off the ground in their communities. You'll find more about the Full Circle America affiliate program in the appendix. But, while I invite all to join with our Full Circle America team, it is less important who does it than that it be done.

• twenty •

Closing Thoughts

THIS JOURNEY HAS BEEN INTENSELY PERSONAL.

It's been personal because I have had to question many previous assumptions and reevaluate the teaching and advice that has shaped my entire professional career. It's been personal because I have committed my all-too-limited spare time and money to this effort. Yet, it increasingly felt much too important to stop, regardless of the obstacles. It's been personal because I also played a significant professional role in the lives and eventual passing of my grandmother and my mother, and now in the life of my father.

It is personal because most of my older patients, by now numbering far more than a thousand, have become my friends. When I tally biweekly to monthly visits for the last two years of life, quarterly visits for the preceding five to ten years, and semiannual visits for another decade, and add daily visits for all the hospitalizations for illness and surgery in between, I have often had well over a hundred visits with every one of my patients by the time they die. That total is more contact than most of us have with all but our closest relatives. And the conversations are often far from superficial. The occasions of such encounters demand discussion of hopes and dreams, future and past, success and failure. What happens to them matters. It is very personal stuff.

Of course, I am not alone in this. It comes with the territory of being a doctor. The older patients of many family physicians are very much their extended families. We care deeply about what happens to them. We question whether we handled everything as well as we could have. We experience loss when they die. Through their spirit and their illnesses they have taught us most of what we know. Our legacy demands that we act on their behalf.

Addressing eldercare creatively demands coming to terms with mortality. The optimist in all of us believes our spirit lives on. In a more down-to-earth, practical sense, figuring out how to age successfully is about confronting death and then moving on to focus on living. Most of my older patients are more rational facing these issues than most of the health-care decision makers.

As Woody Allen said so well, "I am not afraid of dying . . . I just don't want to be there when it happens." Fortunately, most of us will only be "actively dying" for several hours to a few days. I have witnessed probably a thousand deaths and can honestly say there is no reason to fear end-of-life pain or suffering as much as we do. Adequate medication is nearly always available.

During my residency training twenty-five years ago, I participated in two very different end-of-life scenarios. As one of the interns in a 500-bed hospital, I was required to attend, assist, and all too soon run all the "code blues" or cardiac-arrest resuscitative efforts that took place on my shifts. Since this was in the days before living wills were used frequently, hardly a night went by when there were not a few such "codes." Doing CPR and administering lots of medications to a whole army of frail elders, usually without any family or friends even nearby, was a recurring lesson in futility and illogical inhumanity. I have a blended image of so many aged physical bodies without any idea most of the time who they were, or what their lives were about. When I called their families to say that their loved one had died, I hardly ever had any personal connection to them either. It was an institutional death at its worst. Fortunately, that scenario is in the distant past and rarely happens anywhere today.

Also during my residency, I was fortunate to have other very different deaths to attend. As part of our second year of training, one at a time, the residents staffed a small medical clinic overnight in a rural suburban setting twenty miles from the hospital. During my first solo overnight, I was called by a patient's family to come pronounce a just-deceased elder. Driving there in the rain, I nervously reviewed what I needed to do. I was greeted by the son and escorted into the front parlor. To my surprise, this family had converted their spacious formal sitting room into the terminal-care setting for the matriarch of the family.

At least twenty-five family and friends of all ages were seated around the periphery of the room. Well-behaved children were playing on the large hooked rug in the center of the room. The lighting was subdued. Music was quietly playing. In the far corner of the room was a stylish antique twin bed with the deceased woman nestled in a large number of oversized pillows and covered by an Amish quilt. I was stunned and, frankly, totally unprepared for this scene. Thankfully, with my prior elementary-school teaching experience, there was a ready solution right in front of me. I asked a couple of the kids playing on the floor to help me, and I brought them with me to their great-grandmother's bedside.

I then carefully and simply explained to them what I was doing, what had likely happened, and asked them to tell me about her. It more than broke the ice. It led me through a warm introduction to this complete stranger, and gave me the necessary foils to play off of. If only I could be so lucky all the time. What followed was a brief and respectful discussion with the son, a call to the funeral home, and I was off. Now, that family had it all together. All I had to do was pay attention.

And so it has been with pursuing elder alternatives in our small town. Once we get past this overwhelming fear of the unknown, and just jump into doing what needs to be done, the rest is easy. The pieces of the puzzle that must be rearranged to reform elder-care are intimidating, but none of them are very complicated. Like assembling any jigsaw puzzle, you start in one place guided by what makes the most sense, or often just trial and error. Putting a few pieces together leads to a strategy for other sections. Little by little the whole picture comes together. There is nothing intrinsically difficult, but it does require time on task. It does require patience. It does require paying attention.

Never before have so many lived so long in relative good health. Modern science and public-health strategies have made long life the norm. However, societal attitudes and infrastructure have not kept pace with these changes, and the aging of our population is a new phenomenon that requires an entirely new approach, and demands it urgently. The cost of eldercare as we know it will not only bankrupt all our public and private assets, but it will also swamp all the human resources and capacity of our counties, our states, and the entire United States by 2030. The currently available elder options are often undesirable, and deprive us all of one of our richest resources: the wisdom, experience, and friendship of our elders. We cannot rely on the government for solutions. We must rely on each other.

Residential care has become frighteningly complicated and institutional. Nursing homes were never intended to be the primary social support and care option for the vast majority of our elders. They got there by default. They expanded from being a small base for a few older individuals who had fallen through the cracks due to extenuating circumstances to becoming the unavoidable choice for most who live long enough.

Assisted-living facilities came along as a response to the inadequacies of nursing homes to meet the needs of many aging individuals. But the massive number and breadth of this elder cohort—ranging from those one small step away from independent living at home to those one equally small step away from a nursing-home level of need—challenges every ALF administrator and staff member. One size cannot possibly fit all of these older individuals. When we add a regulatory environment borrowed from the highly concentrated medical-care model of the hospital and nursing home world to govern this newer entity, the result is equally untenable. These regulations cannot adequately address the basic elder need for human touch, meaning, and personalized living.

It is into this landscape that the Maine Approach steps. Fortunately, the diversity of individuals' personal homes and their varied interests, talents, and goals provide a rich substrate for a new paradigm. With current technology and a new attitude, an infinitely personalized support system can accommodate this tremendous diversity. There are many moving parts to the new model we've experimented with in Maine and that is laid out in these pages, but the complexity becomes manageable when one considers each piece by itself. We've founded Full Circle America to empower thousands of community-based affiliates to involve, coordinate, and serve the elders of their area through a new model that is dramatically decentralized and with a digital spine holding it together.

All along, the older individuals I've known have shown me the way. They have shared their lives with me. They entrusted me with personal information. They told me brief stories about this or that chapter of their lives. The encounters were unfortunately too short: perhaps a few minutes at the beginning of a medical office visit. But they let me see into their being. Often because I took the time to inquire about the rest of their lives, when the going got tough, they trusted me to help them address the problem. These interludes were not just small talk. "Still skiing 100 days a winter at Sunday River?" "Still flying your ultralight since your heart transplant?" "What grew well in your garden this year?" "Have you had the grandkids here this summer?" The ensuing conversations told me a lot about their current physical and mental health.

These snapshots of their lives and how they told them guided us in conceiving Full Circle America's new paradigm for eldercare. Our model is simply trying to honor, replicate, and systematize what a vast cohort of elders have already proven works. It is so simple, it is revolutionary. We can, as a health-care community, as an enlightened local community, as a network of families and friends, provide the environment that those that we care about desire.

What should be so hard about aiming for a solution that makes those that we care about happy? When that solution is enormously cheaper and has profound positive spin-offs for nearly everyone else, widespread consensus should be a no-brainer.

I owe it to the hundreds of elders who have been patient with me to do no less. I have watched many older individuals graciously accept much less than desired from their assisted-living stay, their nursing home stay, from the medical system in general. It is not that their medical problems were so overwhelming, but that those parts of the system that we all control, that we condone, were falling far short of what these older individuals deserved. So that their energies and the end of their lives will not have been spent in vain, we must seize this golden opportunity to remake our communities, with our elder relatives, friends, and neighbors as an integral part of that rebirth.

It is time to say goodbye to any elder being alone and invisible. Gram Teel would have wanted it that way, and to do any less is foolish.

The Full Circle America Approach

FOR ANYONE INTERESTED IN LEARNING more about Full Circle America or becoming an affiliate, the pages that follow deliver the basics of our program, our structure, and our goals. Further information is available online at www.fullcircleamerica.com—including detailed overviews of affiliate operations, job descriptions, protocols, and eldercare packages.

What Is Full Circle America, Inc.?

- A limited-profit organization that sponsors, trains, supports, and mentors individuals and organizations across the United States seeking to meet the care and lifestyle needs of the elder population in their communities.
- Affiliation with Full Circle America is a unique collaboration. Our primary mission is to support elders in living in the comfort of their homes and in living their lives to the fullest. This is an alternative to assisted living and nursing homes.
- The Full Circle America approach utilizes technology, social networking, life management, and expansive volunteering to accomplish its mission in an affordable way.
- A critical point of difference between Full Circle America and other options is the emphasis upon volunteerism and the inclusion of elders in the

community as an untapped volunteer resource. There are hundreds of thousands of available hours in the retiree community, and every Full Circle America member is encouraged to contribute.

- Full Circle America affiliates must embrace and live the philosophy that our older neighbors are not a burden, but a treasure.

We Are Looking for 10,000 Community Leaders

- Full Circle America seeks affiliate pioneers who can be entrepreneurs, nonprofit organizations, medical groups, and others who embrace the elders of their community, and are comfortable promoting the Full Circle America approach.
- The ideal local promoters are likely to be primary-care physicians' offices, home health agencies, nonprofit agencies, and mature social service organizations. Any of these enterprises may wish to expand the services they offer to area elders.
- Qualified and committed individuals, including, for example, disabled veterans, can also establish a Full Circle America affiliate in their community.
- An ideal affiliate founder should be able to quickly identify at least ten potential members to refer and then enroll in Full Circle America services by the end of the first month. Given the demand for the services rapid growth thereafter is expected.
- A typical, fully mature affiliate will average 100 members.

What Does the Local Full Circle America Affiliate Do?

- Your affiliate Full Circle America will be a stand-alone entity 100 percent locally managed and owned.

- Exactly how your local effort is to be organized is up to the community promoters. To control legal costs, template ownership agreements and bylaws are provided through the National Full Circle America support office.
- The affiliate assumes principal responsibility and authority for the proper delivery of services to its members. It is responsible for recruiting and enrollment of members, equipment installation and maintenance, recruiting and scheduling volunteers, and either hiring or subcontracting for personal support services. It is responsible for recording services rendered, sending invoices, managing accounts payable and accounts receivable.
- The affiliate is licensed to use the Full Circle America trademark and to provide an approved minimum array of services in bundled plans.
- To fully perform its mission, the local affiliate must also coordinate with each member and his or her volunteer team a schedule of life-enriching activities. How this is accomplished is a function of local leadership and the ability to inspire and encourage family, neighbors, schools, religious organizations, and other seniors to participate in the effort.
- The affiliate sets its own prices, collects the membership dues and add-on service fees, and submits a per-member services fee to the national Full Circle America office. Billing services provided through the national FCA office are available.

What Does the National Full Circle Organization Do?

- The National Full Circle organization provides a turnkey operation for its affiliates.

- Training is provided to your manager at no cost through online preparation and a three-day intensive live curriculum. We provide all course materials, lodging, meals, and up to $500 for reimbursement of travel expenses.
- Approved affiliate candidates, with managers who have completed their training, may access an interest-free seed-capital loan to help get them started. No individual will be asked to guarantee this loan, but it will have to be repaid within one year so the funds can be recycled to other new affiliates. The Full Circle national office makes this investment to eliminate a barrier to success, as a vote of confidence in the product and the affiliate, and to help the organization grow as quickly as possible to achieve the mission.
- We provide 24/7 live support, 24/7 remote monitoring surveillance, a comprehensive online operations manual with all the forms necessary for the entire process, complete technology packages ready for easy installation, an easy-to-navigate secure information-technology platform for affiliate and member use, scheduling modules, bookkeeping and accounting software, as well as a commitment to continued product and process development and enhancement.
- Marketing materials and templates will be available online that can be printed locally and distributed in full color.
- In time, the national office will also provide discounted insurance products through a captive insurance company that will offer policies specifically designed to insure the activities of the national and local affiliates.

Steps to Qualify and the Path to Operational Status

- Read all of the materials available online about Full Circle America, along with this book.
- Complete and submit the application form.
- Arrange a telephone interview with principal promoter(s) at Full Circle America.
- Nominate your affiliate manager. Some level of medical or social work experience is recommended but not essential. Full Circle National will conduct a credentials review and telephone interview of the candidate.
- Once the affiliate manager candidate is approved they complete the online training course and then the Full Circle National live-training course, which will be three full days and offered at least monthly.
- The training curriculum will focus on (*a*) attitude toward elders; (*b*) products and program components; (*c*) IT platform and data entry; and (*d*) membership process from recruiting, intake, planning, maintenance, and adjustments to troubleshooting.
- Once the manager has successfully completed training the local affiliate can be organized as an independent entity, and can formally become a Full Circle at-home affiliate. Full Circle National reserves the right to revoke any affiliate license for behavior or practices inconsistent with the Full Circle America brand or mission.
- Once your bank account and EIN have been established and assistance is requested, the national office will wire to the account a nonrecourse no-interest loan to be repaid within one year. A nonrecourse loan is one made to the affiliate and not personally guaranteed by the principal(s).

- Five complete member-technology kits will be provided on consignment to the new affiliate. When a new member is enrolled one of these kits will be immediately installed in his or her home to get started. Enrollment will trigger an invoice to the affiliate that must be paid within ninety days. Even before payment a replacement kit will be shipped to the affiliate in order to assure that the affiliate always has an inventory on hand.
- A fully operational affiliate will have an average of 100 members and will generate sufficient revenue to meet all of its obligations with a reasonable profit available to the investors in the affiliate. FCA cash flow analysis and spread sheets indicate that the break even point for each local affiliate should be between 10 and 25 members and can be achieved in 6–12 months. If the affiliate is a not-for-profit, its fees to members can be reduced, or it can use any surplus to subsidize the needs of those unable to pay for the services.

NOTES

Introduction

1. Shoshana Zuboff, "Our Health-Care System Needs a Bypass," *Bloomberg Businessweek*, Viewpoint, January 16, 2009, p. 1; www.businessweek.com.

Chapter 3

1. Carole Haber, "Nursing Homes: History," http://medicine.jrank.org/pages/1243/Nursing-Homes-History.html.
2. From the booklet "The Story of the Lincoln Home," written in the 1960s.
3. The Online NewsHour, "Timeline—Nursing Homes in America," www.pbs.org.

Chapter 6

1. Rebecca Costa, *The Watchman's Rattle: Thinking Our Way Out of Extinction* (New York: Vanguard Press, 2010), 217–228.

Chapter 16

1. Dorothy Sauber, *Changing Expectations/Planning for the Future: A Parent Advocacy Manual* (Minneapolis: Association for Retarded Citizens Minnesota, 1989).
2. Robert Perske, *Hope for the Families: New Directions for Parents of Persons with Retardation or Other Disabilities* (Nashville, TN: Abingdon Press, 1981).
3. Chris Lyons, "Self-Determination: 'Dignity of Risk'," video and text available on website of The Minnesota Governor's Council on Developmental Disabilities, www.mnddc.org.
4. Stories told by Carolyn Swanson, in article "The Dignity of Risk" published in The Greater Hartford Association for Retarded Citizens, Inc. newsletter, Winter, 2000.
5. Ibid.

Chapter 18

1. Francine Russo, "When Elder Care Brings Back Sibling Tensions," *TIME* February 01, 2010, www.time.com.
2. Jonathan Rausch, "Letting Go of My Father," the *Atlantic*, April 2010, www.theatlantic.com.

ABOUT THE AUTHOR

Allan S. Teel, MD, is a family physician in Damariscotta, Maine. During his twenty-five-year medical career, he has worked with thousands of senior citizens in the hospital, at nursing homes, in assisted-living homes, and in their own homes. Each one has left a lasting impression. Dr. Teel's passion and commitment have driven him to speak out forcefully on the eldercare crisis facing our communities and our country.

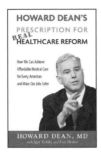
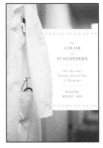
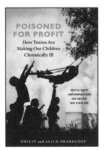
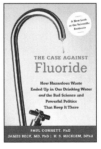
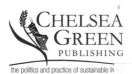
3 1901 05000 3633